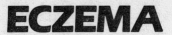
ECZEMA

A comprehensive and objective review of all the options available to sufferers of all ages in the treatment of eczema, plus sound and compassionate advice on avoiding problems while making the most of everyday life.

Paki —
Who knows?
After reading this
book you might be
swearing by "snake-
skin pi-oos"
Here's to your health!

Love,
Thalia
9/21/91

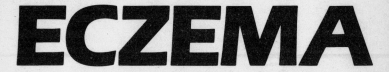

ECZEMA

A Complete Guide to _all_ the Remedies~ Alternative and Orthodox

Christine Orton

THORSONS PUBLISHING GROUP
Wellingborough · New York

First published 1986

British Library Cataloguing in Publication Data

Orton, Christine
   Eczema: a complete guide to the remedies.
   1. Eczema — Treatment
   I. Title
   616.5'21069   RL251

ISBN 0-7225-1180-9

Printed in Great Britain by
Richard Clay (The Chaucer Press) Ltd,
Bungay, Suffolk

Contents

Introduction

This book is the result of a lifetime's experiences of eczema — my son, Adam's. I wish that we had known nineteen years ago when he was born what we know today, and that there had been then the more understanding, accepting and questing attitude to alternative methods of treating this skin condition that there is now.

When he was a baby there were really only steroid preparations to resort to, and even special diets were looked upon as a little cranky and probably pointless, let alone the idea of experimenting with homoeopathy, herbalism and acupuncture. It took courage and great conviction to try alternatives in those days.

In this book I use the description 'alternative' in its widest sense, not just meaning the various therapies of complementary or natural medicine, but any alternatives to the steroid treatments which remain the commonest form of medical management.

From our experiences, and from my personal and professional involvements with the National Eczema Society, I know that many people seek these alternatives. Sometimes we need to use the precribed ointments and creams for short periods of time. But, worried by side-effects and possible dependency, we all want to find ways of resorting to these preparations as little as possible, if at all.

Even so, information on alternative methods of treatment still tends to be scattered and hard to discover. Which is why it seemed to me a useful thing to put everything I already knew, or could find out from others, between two covers. The options are then readily available and what each patient and family does next is up to individual needs and circumstances.

I mention the needs and circumstances of the individual because, as will be clear from every chapter if not every page of this book, eczema is a very individual condition. What helps one will not necessarily help another. The disorder also fluctuates so that it is sometimes severe, sometimes mild, and sometimes quite magically disappears for no apparent reason.

In one way this, of course, is very comforting news. Every eczema sufferer lives with the knowledge that in time the condition may improve, and in certain studies 90 per cent of children with infantile eczema have improved as they grew older.

On the other hand this fluctuation of the disorder does make it difficult to assess progress when trying a new treatment. This is probably one of the main reasons why doctors tend to be very sceptical of improvements when various alternative treatments are tried, often maintaining that the skin would have cleared up anyway.

Sometimes this may be true, but often it has been shown not to be, particularly when a new diet is successful and then old foods are tried again and back comes the rash.

Nevertheless, as yet there is no instant cure for everyone, and in some cases the best that can be done is to keep the symptoms under control until the day does come when the eczema improves of its own accord. Each person has to find his or her own answers, sometimes with the help of doctors and practitioners, and sometimes without.

Because of the wide age group involved, I have written this book for everyone — children with eczema, the people who look after them, the teenage patient, the adult patient. I do not pretend to be an expert, and in many instances am simply reporting as a journalist the experiences and knowledge of others, both patients and practitioners.

I would like to express my warmest thanks to all those who have provided this information and without whose help I certainly could not have managed. In particular I would like to thank Dr David Atherton, paediatric dermatologist with the Great Ormond Street Hospital, not only for his assistance with this book, but also for seeing our family, like a lot of others, through many a crisis with his understanding and enlightened approach.

I should also like to thank the various practitioners of the natural therapies for supplying such helpful information, especially Ray Hill and Thomas Bartram who generously sent pages of practical advice on naturopathy and herbalism.

Another enormous thank you must go to the National Eczema Society for allowing me to quote at great length from its literature and from the quarterly magazine *Exchange*. The NES address, along with those of many other helpful organizations and sources of advice, is given at the end of the book.

Another big thank you to the patients and parents of children with eczema who kindly took the time to supply me with case histories of their own experiences. In doing so they give valuable insight into how treatments mentioned actually work, and bring the book, quite literally, to life.

Finally, yet again, I would like to thank Adam. He, like many others with eczema, has often questioned: 'Why me?' Even if it doesn't always bring much comfort to him, I would like him to be sure that his years of suffering have led to the comfort of thousands of others, originally through the formation of the National Eczema Society and now, I hope, as a result of this book.

For me, writing it has in itself been a learning process. Perhaps we, too, will gain new help in coping with and maybe clearing the condition.

CHRISTINE ORTON

Signs and Symptoms

Though most people think of eczema as just one skin disorder there are, in fact, many types. Even so, there are certain basic symptoms shared by all which give eczema its distinctive appearance and feel — and, as anyone knows who has suffered from the condition or is close to someone who has, these are not at all pleasant to experience.

Seven-year-old Tessa writing about her eczema says: 'Having eczema is not very nice because you keep on scratching and it hurts, and your clothes stick to you.

'And sometimes my legs are so dry I just cannot straighten them. And at night, night always seems worse than daytime. And sometimes I have a bad night's sleep so that means I am very tired and I do not want to go to school next morning.

'I have had eczema since I was 5 weeks old, but hope I will grow out of it one day. Some days I feel very depressed . . .'

Although still so young, Tessa touches on everything that makes eczema so distressing for the patient — the scratching, the disturbed sleep and the subsequent feelings of anxiety and depression.

She also lists the three symptoms which sum up eczema for most people — sore rash, dry skin and itchiness. Even though I've put them in that order, it's hard to know which of these equally upsetting aspects to put first, as each symptom leads to the other and back again. For instance, is the rash caused by the itch and consequent scratching, or is it the other way round? Or is the itchiness itself a result of the dryness of the skin?

No-one has found the answers to these questions yet, as they haven't to many of the mysteries of this skin condition. But I'll start with describing the rash, because this is the outward and visible sign of whatever is causing the inward and hidden disturbance to the normal functioning of the skin.

The rash

Eczema takes its name from the Greek verb 'to boil' which is a good description of the patient's pimply, red rash, often erupting into blistered, weeping and sore patches, particularly after scratching.

The extent of the rash will vary from person to person. For some it may be limited to small areas behind knees or elbows, or show itself on hands, neck and feet. On others, particularly the severe cases, it may occasionally cover the whole body.

The rash will also fluctuate, so that sometimes it is more widespread than others. Doctors tend to think this is because of the capricious, unpredictable nature of the illness, which can also completely disappear, for no apparent reason.

But others would see this coming and going of the rash as cause and effect, even if we do not actually recognize many of the causes as yet. What may seem like chance could be due to some change in lifestyle, of which the person concerned is not even aware.

It could be different diet, a move to a new district where the water is softer, the sudden lifting of a hidden anxiety, sunshine, lack of sunshine, cool winds, a hot climate. There are so many possibilities and so many imponderables — but much more about this in later chapters.

The rash will vary according to the type of eczema — for instance in *discoid* it will be in circular patches, and in the *seborrhoeic* types the rash will affect scalp, face and the hairier areas of the body.

It is the rash, of course, that is the signal to the world that a person has eczema and, quite apart from the physical discomforts, it is the main cause of the emotional and social distress a sufferer can feel.

A rash obviously doesn't look attractive and, perhaps because of infectious illnesses such as measles and chickenpox, even nowadays there are those who think eczema is catching. It is not, but it does lead others to shy away and be wary of touching.

If anything, it is the person with eczema who is vulnerable and not the other way round. Even though eczema is not infectious it can be infected, and this can lead to changes in the appearance of the rash as we'll see in a minute.

Dry skin

The next very common symptom of all types of eczema is an extremely dry skin. Lubricating and moisturizing are becoming the first priority of good treatment because, once the skin is softer and more comfortable, then the rash and irritation are less of a problem, too.

The dryness may also be the first symptoms to show itself when a baby with eczema is born. There may be dry patches on the cheeks and chin, or on elbows and knees. The scalp may also be very dry, looking like a bad case of cradle cap.

As time goes by, and if the eczema develops, the dryness may become so extreme that the skin actually cracks open, particularly at the joints or at any point on the body where the skin is stretched tightly. This can cause a great deal of pain and discomfort, and can often make it difficult for the person to walk or even talk.

Normally our skin is kept supple by oils from the sebaceous glands. These open into the hair follicles and secrete sebum which lubricates both hair and skin. When someone has eczema this process does not run smoothly, and it is necessary to add oil and moisture to the skin, inwardly and outwardly.

With normal skin, the dead cells on the surface are renewed every 28 days or so, and the shedding of the old scales is hardly noticed. But when eczema is severe, the process seems to be speeded up and the flakes are constantly coming away, covering clothes, bedding and even the floor.

This scaling causes all sorts of added problems for the eczema patient. Not only is the dead skin irritating and sometimes embarrassing, it is the food of the dust mite — and this tiny creature is thought to be a common irritant which can trigger or worsen eczema.

So it's important to vacuum regularly, keeping the skin scales as well as the dust mite at bay. Also, the regular use of emulsifiers and moisturizers in the bath and directly on the skin will slow down the scaling and ease the excessive dryness. More of this in the next chapter.

Itchiness

Many consider the itch of eczema to be the worst symptom of all. Even when the rash is hardly visible, the skin can irritate, and the consequent scratching may then bring out the rash and soreness, creating a vicious circle.

One adult patient describes this irritation as being quite different from the sort most of us feel from time to time when we have a gnat bite or some minor skin upset. She calls it the 'Third Degree Itch', unique to eczema sufferers.

'The itch is deep *under* the skin,' she explains. 'It feels like a mass of mosquitoes biting from underneath. The onset is rapid, severe and erratic and the most urgent need is to obtain quick relief by scratching.

'Once pain is experienced, the itch subsides as rapidly as its onset. Pain, of course, hurts — but is sweet relief compared to the itch.'

The writer also describes what she calls 'the burn'. 'The skin feels as if concentrated acid is running through the veins. Burning usually starts before the itch and can be a short forewarning to the rapid onset of Third Degree Itch. The excessive heat is localized and another part of the body may feel quite cold.'

This is an example of the loss of temperature control which affects many people with eczema, probably because the skin surface is so damaged. The sweat pores may also function poorly so that there is little perspiration.

It is thought that the nerve system of the skin which reaches right down to the deeper level of the dermis is sensitive to itch as well as to pain, heat, cold and touch.

Experts believe that people with eczema have a natural tendency to itch and that their threshold to irritation is much lower than that of others. The skin is hyper-sensitive, and what feels like touch to anyone else will be an 'itch' for the eczema sufferer.

Sometimes there seems to be an obvious trigger, such as wool worn next to the skin, or strong washing detergent left on clothes after rinsing. Animal hairs, dust, pollen, grass, plants, certain foods, heat or cold, dryness or wetness, worry, excitement, exercise — all and many more can irritate the sensitive skin.

But at other times there seems to be no traceable reason, and the irritation can just build up gradually or arrive suddenly, as one patient describes it 'like a tropical thunder storm.'

Scratching the itch

The effects of scratching, both on the skin and on the feelings of the sufferer, can be catastrophic. Though children may do it openly, an adult is more likely to hide away, but both end up feeling ashamed and beaten, knowing in the end that the scratching can only make matters worse.

In spite of this, the most helpful attitude towards the scratching is acceptance, both on the part of patients and those close to them. To feel guilty yourself, or to keep telling another person to 'stop scratching' doesn't really help.

In fact, if scratching — or at least rubbing — is allowed then there is likely to be less scratching at night during sleep, when there might otherwise be a build-up of the urge and no conscious control to stop it.

Of course, the irritation is not always inevitable. If there are particular triggers, then perhaps these can be identified and avoided. There are also certain preparations, including antihistamines and homoeopathic and herbal remedies, that can calm irritation and also encourage sleep at night.

Infected eczema

Infection is one of the commonest reasons among children and adults for a sudden worsening of eczema or changes in the appearance of the rash.

If there are yellow pimples or pus-filled blisters, or weeping and crusting of the skin, plus perhaps swollen glands and a slight temperature, then it is likely that eczema has been infected by the same bacteria which causes *impetigo* in ordinary skin.

Another danger is the *herpes simplex virus 1* which in the ordinary person causes cold sores round the mouth, but in children with eczema can trigger off a quite serious illness called *eczema herpeticum*, described on page 24.

Just as the person with a cold sore should never kiss or touch a child with eczema, anyone with a skin infection such as impetigo should steer well clear, too, and not share towels, cups and so on.

If eczema does become infected with bacteria it is unlikely to cause the havoc that eczema herpeticum can, but still needs careful treatment. Antiseptics and antibiotics play a useful part, as do some more traditional methods such as painting with antiseptic dyes or using homoeopathic or herbal remedies. Steroid preparations should not normally be prescribed when infection is diagnosed, although some do have an antibiotic added. Some of these will have the letter A, C or M after the brand name.

When smallpox was still rife, this presented extra problems for anyone with eczema visiting a foreign country, since smallpox vaccination could also cause a virus called *eczema vaccinatum*.

Nowadays, since smallpox has been more or less eradicated, this difficulty for travellers with eczema no longer presents itself, but it is still necessary to take care with all types of immunization.

Though doctors no longer see eczema as a reason for not being immunized, if a child is suffering from very severe eczema then it would seem best to postpone any jabs. Also, if there is a very pronounced allergy to chicken or eggs, some vaccines may be unsuitable.

So the fact that a child, or an adult going abroad and needing immunization, has eczema should always be made clear to doctor or clinic before any action is taken.

Social effects

Another aspect of eczema that is shared by all those who have this condition, regardless of type, is the sense of stigma that so often seems to go with skin disorders.

Though there are times when this can be imagined, and is more in the mind of the sufferer than in the eye of the beholder, there is no doubt that occasionally other people do turn away from the person who has an obvious rash.

I have seen this with my own son, when people at swimming pools have stared outrageously at his sore skin, and even stopped in their tracks and turned round to take a second look when it has been particularly bad.

At school, like many other children with eczema, he was called names such as 'spotty' and 'flaky', and even at one time 'ET'. Although now he is older he has many good friends, there was a time when he found it very difficult to get close to anyone, physically as well as emotionally.

It's a problem that many people with skin disorders come up against and find as difficult to bear as the physical symptoms. As one young women of twenty-seven says: 'If you see someone in a wheelchair, or someone who is blind, you show them sympathy and kindness. But people react differently towards skin complaints. Children and adults alike will actually move away from you if they happen to sit next to you on the bus or train, and suddenly notice it. How much worse that reaction will make the person feel!'

A part of this, as I've already mentioned, must be because others fear that the rash may be contagious. Not everyone knows that you can't catch eczema like measles — and even if they do they won't necessarily realize that the rash is eczema, anyway.

But unless they have the disorder themselves, or know someone else who has, people are generally very uninformed about eczema, and may have the idea that it is somehow unhygienic or caused through neglect. This is painful for both patient and family, particularly when they are usually trying desperately hard to control the condition and it simply won't go away.

Even so, a great deal can be done to help in this shared difficulty, which I hope will become clear as you read further into this book. The cure is really two-way — by talking openly about the condition and joining forces with others it is possible to educate the public at large about what eczema is and isn't.

By changing mental attitudes within themselves, those who have eczema and those who look after them may become more confident and better able to cope with other people. Who knows, by changing attitudes that rash might even go away!

Nerves and eczema

Having said that, I would like to deny the existence of what some doctors have been known to call 'nervous eczema.'

It's true that there are mentally ill people who purposely damage their skin or intentionally eat foods or use harmful substances to trigger off a rash. There is also a condition called *lichen simplex* when a rash will form if someone nervously and repeatedly scratches a particular area, for instance the neck.

It's also true that stress and anxiety may play a part in causing or worsening eczema, but this is only one of many factors which will act as a trigger, including heredity, diet, allergy and sensitivity in general, cell formation and skin type.

To be told that eczema is 'all nerves' is usually uninformed rubbish, and very frustrating both for the person suffering from the condition and for parents. It is far more likely that the physical discomforts and spoilt appearance cause anxiety and depression than the other way round.

All this is explored in greater depth, with some solutions, in Chapter 12. But both the emotional and social effects of eczema are so profound and such an integral part of the disorder, that I wanted to state my case on this important aspect right at the beginning.

This mistaken attitude over the connections between emotion and eczema can even lead to mis-diagnosis and the prolonging of the illness. The case of twenty-six-year-old Sandra, quoted in *Exchange*, the National Eczema Society magazine, is a typical example.

Sandra had always suffered from eczema, which her doctor and family put down to 'nerves'. Then one summer a rash developed over most of her body. She was prescribed *Valium*, a tranquillizer, and was put on a course of systemic steroids.

'The relief was unbelievable,' she writes. 'I thought I was cured, not to know that this was the start of months more agony and heartbreak. Everytime the steroids were reduced slightly the rash came back worse than ever and over the weeks the steroids became less effective.

'I have never really bothered that my hands were clear, and also my legs below the knees, until one day I stood in front of the mirror looking at the mess I was in and realized my neck was clear, also the V of the neckline and my cleavage.

'I wondered if it was the fabric softener that I used, so all my clothes were rewashed, but to no avail. The next thing I did was to wash some clothes in pure soap and within 3 days there was scarcely a sore in sight. I could hardly believe that after all this time my skin was showing some improvement.'

Sandra's skin was so damaged by the steroid treatment that it remained very sensitive, but she found she could get by just using cold cream. Best of all, her doctor booked her into the local hospital for allergy tests and stopped prescribing tranquillizers.

What's the Type?

It is very important to have eczema correctly diagnosed, because management and treatment will vary according to type. What suits one may not necessarily suit another, and in some cases may even make things worse.

There are thought to be around fourteen different sorts of eczema, and the following are among the most common.

Atopic eczema

This is particularly widespread among babies and young children, which is why *atopic eczema* is also called *infantile eczema*. Though most children clear as they grow older, atopic eczema can continue through adolesence and into adulthood.

Atopic eczema is thought to be an inherited tendency and patients often have *hayfever, rhinitis* and *asthma* as well, or have a relative who suffers from one of these allied illnesses. So, when deciding whether a child's eczema is atopic, it often helps to take a look at the family tree.

Another useful point is that the skin of the atopic differs from other people's. It is generally paler, though areas may become red and inflamed because the underlying blood vessels are dilated and near the surface. But if you run a finger across the skin, it will whiten at the point of contact.

Even though most eczema sufferers have a dry and sensitive skin the atopic's tends to be excessively so, and is generally very sensitive. When eczema does clear the complexion can be exceptionally fine, rather like a young baby's.

What triggers off atopic eczema is not certain. Although asthma and hayfever are known to be strongly allergic conditions, whether or not atopic eczema is a straightforward allergic reaction has not been definitely proved.

Certainly special diets and avoidance of irritants can make a difference, but reactions are individual and not everyone is helped in this way. Another problem can be that the atopic is sensitive to so many things that it is almost impossible to avoid them all.

One theory is that the immune system of the atopic, which protects against allergy, is late in developing and this is perhaps why, as they grow older, children often grow out of their eczema.

It may also explain why babies born of 'at risk' parents in families where someone already has eczema, asthma or hayfever, stand less chance of developing the condition if they are kept away from the most common allergy provokers such as cow's milk, eggs and wheat for the first months of life.

There is still a great deal to be discovered about atopic eczema, but meanwhile many parents and adult patients are finding that, by experimenting carefully with diet and with various forms of alternative treatments, they can successfully control the eczema, and sometimes clear it completely.

Contact eczema

If children mainly suffer from atopic eczema, among adults *contact eczema* is one of the most common types to be found. This can either be caused by an irritant which damages the skin's surface (*irritant contact eczema*) or by a substance actually penetrating the skin and setting up an allergic reaction (*allergic contact eczema*).

As Dr John Burton explains in his excellent book *Essentials of Dermatology*, a primary irritant is a substance which, if applied in high enough concentration to normal skin, is capable of producing eczema. Caustic liquids such as acids and alkalis are a good example of this, but milder irritants can be the ingredients of washing powders and washing-up liquids, or mineral oils, chemicals and solvents.

Allergic contact eczema, on the other hand, only develops in someone who has become sensitive — or allergic — to that particular substance. Common allergens are metals, especially nickel and chromium. These are found in jewellery, but also in less obvious things such as detergent and cement.

Also common are rubbers, organic dyes, plastic and resins (as used in spectacles and nail varnish), preservatives in ointments and cosmetics, plants (especialy primula) and drugs applied to the skin (especially antihistamines).

Because many of these allergens are found in factories or working life generally, this type of eczema is often called *industrial eczema*. The term *dermatitis* is also used, which can be confusing because people think of it as a separate skin condition. In fact eczema and dermatitis are one and the same.

If contact eczema is suspected, then patch testing can be used to find out what may be causing the trouble. After discussion about possible suspects, minute amounts of various substances are placed against the skin for 48 hours. If a rash or redness develops in that area then the patient will try and avoid the cause in future.

There can be difficulties in detecting a possible offender. For instance, though the rash may develop at the point of contact, this may not always be the case, and a secondary rash may develop some way from the original contact. Also, sensitivity to a substance can take a long time to develop.

So a woman who has been wearing rubber gloves or a nickel bracelet for years may not connect her new rash with either of these. And when sensitivity to a nail varnish causes a rash on chin or eyelids you can easily forget how often the hands touch the face.

It can also be very difficult avoiding certain irritants and allergens, particularly if they are involved in your livelihood or daily chores at home. Occasionally the problem may mean a change of job, although more often protective clothing or a switch in routine may do the trick.

If the contact eczema disappears, then most people will agree it is worth making some effort, and this is certainly one of the types of eczema where there is a high chance of complete recovery.

Seborrhoeic eczema
Seborrhoeic eczema, which affects both very young babies and adults, can be confusing because, particularly in babies, it may be mistaken for atopic eczema. The big difference is that it often clears up quickly.

At around three months of age the baby of Jane, a friend of mine, developed thick scaling on his scalp which looked like cradle cap, and a rash started moving down his face and onto his body.

The doctor prescribed steroid preparations, but as soon as Jane stopped using these on her baby the rash spread further. We discussed the possibility of seborrhoeic eczema and she started bathing him using emulsifying ointment instead of soap and abandoned the hydrocortisone and other steroid preparations altogether.

Jane also treated the scaly scalp with olive oil, a gentle tar shampoo and an old-fashioned preparation called *Pickles SRN* which gently lifted the dry scales away.

Lo and behold, within a matter of months his head and body were completely clear and the rash has never returned. This would seem to be a clear example of seborrhoeic eczema, and it's frightening to think what might have happened had this baby been caught on the treadmill of unnecessary steroid preparations.

The symptoms are very similar in adults, usually starting with a scaly scalp and bad dandruff, and developing into a rash which can move down the forehead, round the nostrils, behind the ears, upper back and chest and even trunk. The term seborrhoeic is not really understood, except that the eczema appears to affect the hairier parts of the body.

The best treatment for adults seems to be to sort the scalp out first, using special shampoos — for instance, one like *Polytar* — to soothe the skin and clear the dandruff. Very often the rash will then clear, too, but if it returns again simply follow the same routine.

If the rash is persistent then anti-yeast creams prescribed by the doctor could be helpful, or follow the advice given in later chapters for alternative ways of managing all types of eczema.

Pompholyx eczema

Pompholyx is a type of blistering eczema which only affects the palms of hands and soles of feet, although it can be combined with other types of eczema affecting other parts of the body.

Writes Vera, now in her fifties: 'About nineteen years ago I noticed a peculiar formation of tiny red spots on the palm of my right hand. They formed perfect tiny circles about 3 mm in diameter.

'The spots grew from the size of a pinhead to a small blister, which burst. All the time the skin was incredibly dry and hard. My hand would split into deep cuts which would then bleed, and was very painful. The skin was thick and hard, and I could peel it off quite easily to reveal a most unhealthy looking layer of skin underneath.'

Once again, this type of eczema can be confused with similar looking disorders — in this case *athlete's foot* — and it's essential to know which is which as treatments, particularly medical ones, will be quite different. Steroid preparations, for instance, will make a fungal infection like athlete's foot spread rather than subside.

It is thought that overheating is often a trigger for pompholyx eczema, which is why many cases erupt in summer. Nylon socks, rubber-soled footwear and rubber gloves should also be avoided, and potassium permanganate soaks can ease the discomfort and irritation.

Light-sensitive eczema

Many people find that their eczema is helped by sunshine, but others discover that the rash is actually caused, or at any rate made worse, by being exposed to the light. They have to wear a barrier cream and protective clothing and may even have to avoid going out of doors.

Light-sensitive eczema is fairly rare and tends to affect men over forty, although women are also occasionally affected. There are various forms of the sensitivity, and these include *chronic actinic dermatitis, photo-sensitive eczema* and *actinic reticuloid.*

Drugs and cosmetics can also increase sensitivity to light and special skin allergy tests called photopatch tests are carried out, as well as light tests, to try and pinpoint the cause.

In a few people atopic eczema and seborrhoeic eczema can also be light-sensitive, so that the rash becomes worse some hours after being exposed.

In all these types of light-sensitive eczema it is ultra-violet light which causes most of the trouble. This is strongest when the sun is highest in the sky, that is, in the middle of the day, but can also be there in cloudy, hazy or quite cool weather.

It is obviously very important to have this particular type of eczema diagnosed, as a great deal can be done to help the problem once the source is discovered.

Discoid and varicose eczemas

These are two more types of eczema which tend to affect middle-aged and elderly people rather than the young. In *discoid eczema* the rash forms into coin shaped patches on the limbs.

In *varicose eczema* (also known as *gravitational* and *statis eczema*) the rash is allied to varicose veins, ulcers and sluggish blood flow, and appears on the lower part of the legs.

The rash can also spread to other parts of the body later, and there can be an allergic reaction to some of the preparations prescribed to treat the condition (for instance antibiotics). So it can be a complicated condition to treat.

Another disorder affecting elderly people is *asteatotic eczema* but this usually results from other illnesses, such as kidney disease, which cause the skin to become dry and flaky. Lubricating and moisturizing creams for the dryness and cracking will often clear up the irritating rash.

Eczema herpeticum

This is not really a type of eczema, but the effect on eczema of infection by the *Herpes Simplex Virus 1* which also causes cold sores on the mouth.

Young children with atopic eczema seem to be especially vulnerable to this particular complication, perhaps because they have not yet built up the necessary bodily defences, and eczema herpeticum can be a serious illness if not promptly and correctly treated.

The virus infection causes the eczema to spread, with small blisters forming filled with first clear liquid, and later pus. These may burst and the rash will become yellow and crusted. The child is likely to have a high temperature, go off food and lose energy.

Usually eczema herpeticum needs prompt hospital care, and there is medical treatment available which will cure the infection quickly. But unfortunately not enough people, doctors included, recognize the condition.

One mother tells the alarming story of a GP who diagnosed her son as having a 'throat infection' when his eczema blistered and he was running a high temperature. The next day they were turned away from a hospital casualty department because the doctor on duty dismissed what in fact was eczema herpeticum as a 'flare-up of the eczema'.

Luckily their son was eventually admitted and recovered after treatment but, as this mother points out, it is no wonder that eczema herpeticum is occasionally fatal when doctors cannot identify the illness.

The National Eczema Society has useful literature on this condition, as on many other aspects and types of eczema, and a copy of the leaflet could be shown to doctors or hospital staff if eczema herpeticum is suspected.

Other disorders

Finally it is, of course, possible to suffer from other skin disorders, side-by-side with the eczema, which confuse diagnosis and treatment.

Urticaria, also known as nettle rash and hives, is the spotty, bumpy rash which many people get as a reaction to anything from a wasp sting to eating strawberries. It is often this, and not the eczema, which breaks out when a particular food is eaten or substance touched.

Even though diet or a change in lifestyle may clear the urticaria and not the eczema, this would still be worthwhile and would ease general discomfort. But just bear in mind that you may be dealing with two separate conditions.

Someone with eczema may also have *ichthyosis,* commonly known as 'fish-scale disease', a rather unkind name which nevertheless does aptly sum up the appearance of the condition. The skin is acutely dry, far more so than with eczema alone, and needs special treatment.

Eczema can occasionally affect the outer parts of the eye, making them sore and itchy. This is called *vernal disease* or spring catarrh, and is treatable. People with atopic eczema can also very occasionally develop cataracts, so any discomfort should be quickly reported to an eye specialist.

There are obviously many other skin rashes which anyone with eczema can have, from *measles* and *chickenpox* to *shingles.* But luckily these do not usually seem to have a worse effect than normal, a fact I can substantiate as our son has had all three, plus *thrush,* fungal infection of the nails and goodness know what else!

Some researchers wonder whether eczema sufferers have a particular vulnerability to all infection, and perhaps the broken skin does make this so on occasion. On the other hand, it is comforting to know that most of the time their resistance is high, emotionally as well as physically.

They soldier on through all sorts of discomforts and torments which would make many people despair. Eczema may not be dramatic, and is not usually life-threatening, but its agonies are like the slow drip-drip of a tap.

As one mother, whose son David has suffered from atopic eczema since he was a few months old, says in praise: 'It never fails to amaze me how patient, brave and optimistic children and adults are when they suffer so much, day in and day out.'

Treating the Skin

Steroid creams and ointments are the most commonly prescribed medical treatment for eczema, and this has been the case for many years now.

When they arrived on the scene thirty or so years ago, these preparations were hailed as the saviours of all eczema sufferers, miraculously healing the rash, itch *and* dry skin. Traditional treatments such as tar and zinc pastes, bandaging and herbal remedies mostly went out of the window.

With the blessing of the medical profession patients applied steroid preparations for every rash, from the mildest to most severe, often using them as lavishly as they would any face cream or body lotion.

It was only gradually that dark rumours of side-effects such as atrophy of the skin and stunting of growth began to filter through, and people began to wonder whether the creams and ointments were so harmless after all. As a specialist writing in *Exchange* describes, any new treatment seems to pass through three distinct stages.

'In the first — the age of discovery — the therapeutic advantages appear to outweigh any possible side-effects and the drug is prescribed for an increasingly wide spectrum of disease.

'In the second — the age of scepticism — doubts are raised as to the drug's efficiency and much more note is taken of side-effects and complications. Finally — in the age of reason — a balanced view is obtained with the advantages of the drug being finely weighed against a background of experience.'

Hidden threat

This, then, should be age of reason as far as the treatment of eczema with steroid preparations goes. Yet many people are more worried than ever, both by the attitude and actions of certain doctors and by the still unclear but possible threat of side-effects.

Basically, the steroids used to treat eczema are laboratory-manufactured hormones which are similar to the cortisol produced naturally by the body to control inflammation. Since eczema is a type of inflammation, it has been found that this artificial cortisol can keep the rash under control.

Hydrocortisone, the weakest of the steroid preparations, is simply cortisol which has been produced in a laboratory. *Betnovate, Locoid, Dermovate* and many other preparations now available are specially formed to be more powerful and may have other ingredients added, including lubricants and antibiotics.

If these preparations are used on the site of the inflammation — that is, the skin — they are called topical steroids. Systemic steroids reach organs in the body through the blood and are given by injection or in tablet form by mouth.

As the specialist already quoted goes on to explain, there are two main problems associated with excess use of steroids — one is the suppression of the body's own steroid glands, called adrenal suppression, and the other is the thinning of the skin, or atrophy.

The suppression of the body's own steroid glands means that the artificial steroids, if absorbed into the bloodstream, might lessen the production of natural cortisol by the body so that if the patient has an infection or shock, such as an operation, there is less resistance.

'Atrophy develops because steroids weaken and lessen the collagen content of the skin which is its basic support protein. This not only affects the top layer of the skin, the epidermis, but also the lower layer of the skin, the dermis.

'The skin can become thinner so that it cracks and blood vessels become more prominent, giving a flushed appearance, particularly to the face. The loss of collagen can also lead to striae, or stretch marks, which are similar in appearance to the stretch marks of pregnancy.

But the first of these side-effects, this specialist says, only becomes a problem when large quantities of a very strong steroid are used over a short space of time. The risk of stretch marks and skin thinning, however, is more complex.

This depends not only on the strength and quantity of steroid used, but also on duration of use and site of application. For instance, one should be especially careful when using steroid preparations on the face, in the body folds or on children.

Research at this specialist's hospital suggests that weak hydrocortisone does not cause skin thinning, but the risk with other steroids varies according to their potency. The stronger the steroid, the more risk of skin thinning.

Even though with the strongest steroid this appears to be reversible in the short term, when used over a period of several years — or even months — then the effects can be permanent.

Unknown precautions

So it seems the safe use of steroids depends on both doctors and the people using the preparations being aware of the possible side-effects and sticking carefully by the rules, using only the weakest preparations for as short a time as possible on less vulnerable areas of the body.

Unfortunately this is all too often not the case, mainly because, whether out of ignorance or carelessness, many doctors and even skin specialists do not pass on the necessary information to their patients.

Every week bundles of letters arrive at the head office of the National Eczema Society showing this. Mothers are still being prescribed medium to strong steroid preparations for their young babies, and adults are receiving repeat prescriptions for the strongest preparations without clear instructions of how or where to put them.

Writes one young woman: 'In my early teens I was prescribed *Propaderm* for my face. I used it for about two to three years, generously applying it every morning. As a result my skin is quite thin on my face. I already have lines around my nose and cheeks and my skin is very dry. My face has become red, blotchy and transparent.

Says another writer: 'I was put on *Synalar* cream by my doctor and I suffered outbreaks of redness and dryness which resulted in a very blotchy skin. The only instructions ever given me were to use twice a day in the morning and the evening.

'I have continued to use this cream ever since as a make-up base and in the quantity you would use a cold cream. I was never aware that it contained cortisone or was a steroid, and was never told to use sparingly.'

The trouble for patients if they are not given proper advice is that, at present, there is no way they can know the dangers from looking at packets or tubes. These bear no indication of strength and very often no further instructions than the brief: 'Apply as directed.'

With new legislation which allows certain preparations to be bought from the chemist, the need for more detailed information has become even greater and the NES leaflet 'Skin Care' lists strengths of steroid preparations.

But even those who have learned about correct application, either from doctors or from the National Eczema Society, still have serious misgivings about using the steroid preparations. Often this is because they are unnecessarily and inappropriately prescribed.

I have already mentioned two cases like this — Jane, whose baby was prescribed strong steroid ointment at a very early age for a condition that would have cleared without it, and Sandra who was on both systemic steroids and transquillizers before it was discovered her eczema was due to washing powder.

Too many GPs seem to rush to prescribe steroids when some other course of treatment could and should be taken. In emergency and after other alternative methods have been tried there is no doubt that steroid preparations can suppress symptoms and ease discomfort, but they should not be the first line of defence.

Hidden effects

Another reason for patients and their families to be wary of steroid use is that, in spite of all the assurances to the contrary, it is not certain that all the facts about side-effects are being made clear.

For instance, doctors have been saying for years that the greater risks lie with systemic steroids taken internally, and that, used sensibly, topical steroids are safe because, of course, they cannot be absorbed through the skin and into the blood-stream.

But recently, when a boy of seventeen was taken into hospitals for specialists to look into his slow rate of growth, blood tests showed that even the weakest hydrocortisone was being absorbed. Reports his mother:

'Our son has been on *Betnovate* and various other strong steroid preparations since he was a baby, including a year on *Dermovate*, the strongest of all. This was before we had any idea about side-effects.

'But even after we did learn, we comforted ourselves with the fact that the preparations could not be absorbed. Then, after the blood-tests, the doctors revealed that when skin was as damaged and thin as our son's, absorption was possible and had probably caused his growth problems. He was the second teenager they had seen that month with the same experience. '

Her son's apparent dependency on the preparations also worries this mother, and like many parents and patients she is concerned that the steroids started at such an early age might have actually perpetuated the condition.

Steroids are known to have a rebound effect, and if stopped suddenly the eczema will become much worse. Patients often notice, too, that after using a preparation on a small patch of eczema, the patch will come back again twice as big. One preparation, *Dermovate*, has been proved actually to *cause* a rash if used round the mouth.

There also seems to be patient evidence that the skin builds up a type of immunity to preparations, so that even if a weaker one is used to start with, stronger and stronger preparations are needed to keep the rash at bay.

The name given to this particular side-effect of some modern drugs is iatrogenic: illness caused by medical treatment. In his book *Diseases of Civilisation* Brian Inglis gives a whole list of these diseases, and includes steroid treatments in all their forms because of the effects they can have.

Topical steroid treatments, he points out, can give short-term relief, but they can also do long-term harm and few manufacturers enclose warnings with their products. If they do, then the chemist is likely to take them out with the excuse that 'it is up to the doctor what to tell the patient.'

I do not wish to alarm and upset people unnecessarily, and we know from our own experience what a Godsend steroid preparations can be. When he was quite young we tried for a whole year to keep Adam off all of them, experimenting instead with diet and herbal remedies.

But he finished that year with two months in hospital, unable to go to school, play football or even walk at times, and we had to give up the battle. Even though we tried to use only the weakest preparations, they allowed him to lead a more normal life with some enjoyment.

Now, though, I sometimes wonder whether this was at the expense of his long term good and once again we are trying alternative methods ourselves, such as ultra-violet light (PUVA), bandages impregnated with tar and, most recently, acupressure and massage.

It's interesting to see that the best GPs and skin specialists are turning to the more traditional methods of soothing the skin and calming the itch. They, too, are concerned about the long-term affects of steroid preparations, particularly among young children, and until these fears have been definitely allayed prefer to keep them to a minimum, or substitute alternatives that are tried, tested and known to be completely safe.

Moisturizing baths

Increasingly doctors are finding that the first priority in the successful treatment of eczema is to lubricate and moisturize the skin to replace lost water and oils, because it is the dryness that causes much of the soreness and irritation.

A surprise to some is that one of the most helpful ways of doing this is by daily baths. Though it is true that water alone can have a drying effect on the skin, and also that many soaps are an irritant and best not used, the right sort of bath can be very beneficial.

This is a bath containing some form of emulsifier or lubricant which locks the water into the skin with a covering of oil. The most popular are oils such as *Alpha Keri* or *Oilatum*, or an emulsifying ointment like *Unguentum Emulsificans*, or a combination of both.

The water should not be too hot, as this will overheat the body and, even though there may be short-term relief, can lead to itchiness and discomfort later. As the bath is running, pour in 15-30 ml of the oil and/or add the emulsifying ointment.

One way of using the emulsifying ointment is to dissolve two tablespoons in a jug of boiling water, stirring or whisking thoroughly and then adding to the bath. Another way is to use the emulsifying ointment as you would a soap, taking a lump from the container and massaging it into the skin all over the body.

For many patients, and parents of children with eczema, this simple treatment has been a turning point in getting to grips with the condition, leading to enormous general improvements. Says Brenda, the mother of two children with eczema, who had previously tried many remedies without success:

'I was very sceptical of success when I discovered that the basis of the new treatment was prolonged and frequent baths to which were added liberal amounts of emulsifying ointment, previously dissolved in hot water.

'Baths, even when using emulsifying ointment, had always been a traumatic experience, to be finished as soon as possible to the relief to one and all. With considerable trepidation at the idea of two 20 minute baths for each child a day, we embarked on the new treatment.

'Since then the twice daily bathing routine has brought about a wonderful improvement in the condition of their skins. Gone are the broken nights and the daily washing of sheets. It is no longer necessary to vacuum the white flakes of skin from the bedroom carpet each morning. At school they have been able to make friends without the handicap of their sore skins.'

The mother of a seven-year-old girl writes: 'Ten days ago we saw a skin specialist regarding her eczema and he gave us what he called 'gunge', which is really emulsifying ointment BP to be used as soap in the bath.

'The result is a miracle — her skin is like a normal child's at last, soft all over with no eczema. I have left off the two creams, hydrocortisone and *Betnovate*, as she doesn't need them. Her bed always used to be a mess with the skin bleeding and dry flakes everywhere, but today the sheets are just ordinary and I felt I must tell you of this wonderful improvement.'

One word of warning — it is possible for the skin to be sensitive to even the most harmless-seeming things, and so any new treatment should be watched carefully for any signs of reaction. For instance, *Alpha Keri* and various other lubricants contain lanolin, to which some people are allergic. If this is the case, switch to some other emulsifier in the bath such as aqueous cream or *Unguentum Merck*, smoothing it into the skin as you would an emulsifying ointment.

Nor are all eczema sufferers sensitive to all soaps, particularly those free from harmful ingredients such as perfume and preservative, usually known as 'hypoallergenic'. Some soaps, such as those made from goat's milk or containing herbs, are especially formulated to soothe sore skins, and *Simple Soap* contains none of the usual irritants.

Another effective and traditional addition to the bath is oatmeal, which forms into particles and adheres to the skin, helping it maintain its water content and soothing soreness. One oatmeal product is in the form of a tablet, like soap, and is called *Aveenobar*. It is also sold in sachet form, either with or without oil.

Ointments and creams

Immediately after baths and as often as possible during the day, emulsifying creams and ointments should be gently massaged into the skin to keep up the moisture content and combat any dryness and cracking.

Whether an ointment or a cream is used is really a matter of personal preference. From a cosmetic point of view, creams (which are suspensions of fat droplets in water) are on the whole less oily and not so obvious on the skin. Ointments (suspensions of water in fat or just fat alone) are heavier and greasier and therefore more noticeable, but do tend to stay on the skin longer.

Choice will also depend on individual skin type. The drier the skin, the greasier the preparation needed to counteract this. But some people simply feel more comfortable with one than the other, and the only way is to experiment.

Another advantage that ointments have over creams, however, is that they are less likely to become contaminated by bacteria and therefore do not have to contain preservatives which can irritate or cause an allergic reaction in the skin.

There are many moisturizing and lubricating preparations available, some of which can be bought across the chemist's counter or from herbalist or homoeopathic suppliers. Others are available on prescription from a GP or skin specialist.

A good choice includes Aqueous cream BP, E45 cream, Oily cream BP, *Aquadrate, Ultrabase, Unguentum Merck,* and white soft paraffin. You can also use emulsifying ointment as a moisturizer in and out of the bath.

There are many more possibilities, and during my years as editor of the NES magazine *Exchange* I have received letters from people who have hit upon all sorts of remedies. Some have been around for years and may not at first have seemed an obvious answer, but have turned out to suit an individual need.

Writes the mother of a young baby: 'My daughter aged fifteen months suffers from severe eczema and her skin has a tendency to dry out in cold weather and bake in hot. We have found that coconut oil, liberally applied, helps to alleviate her suffering and prevent some itching.'

Writes an adult reader: 'The only thing handy was *Nivea* cream. I used this with some anxiety, but by morning the skin seemed less angry so I continued to use it for one week and found the skin seemed softer than ever before. I have tried many different creams, some on prescription and some not, but so far this seems the best.'

Some people recommend *Vaseline*, some the oil from vitamin capsules, some Evening Primrose oil applied direct to the skin as well as taken internally. Others swear by *Jojoba Moisture Cream* which you can find in the chain of Body Shops along with many other natural and herbal remedies.

It can be an expensive process testing individual reactions, but if and when you hit upon the right answer for you, the rewards make up for it.

Medicinal preparations

Many creams and ointments contain additional ingredients which are soothing, healing or anti-itch. For instance, urea is a natural chemical which can attract and keep water in the skin. Research is also continuing on the use of sodium cromoglycate for eczema, a drug which has already been successful in spray form for asthma and hayfever.

Zinc oxide and zinc carbonate are mineral substances which cool the inflamed skin and protect it from irritation, and coal tar is a mixture of chemical substances which also have a soothing effect.

All have been popular in the treatment of eczema for years and are often used in the creams, ointments and pastes prescribed today. Calamine is another good old-fashioned remedy, but it does tend to dry an already over-dry skin. Nor are tars and pastes always so cosmetically pleasant as modern preparations, but at least there is no worry about side-effects.

Writes the mother of Sorrel, a little girl with eczema: '*Lassar's Paste* is apparently a very old remedy, and is also known as paste of zinc and salicylic acid. It contains a lot of powder and is heavy and messy to use and comes off on clothes. But I use it on Sorrel at night, and it has helped her skin considerably after many months of trying assorted creams.'

Care must be taken, however, when trying over-the-counter preparations. For instance, antihistamine creams might sound just the right answer and are, in fact, useful for treating urticaria after wasp stings, gnat bites and so on. But they are not suitable for eczema and may even cause an allergic reaction and make the rash worse.

All wrapped up

Before the era of steroid treatments it was common practice to bandage children with severe eczema, partly to keep creams and ointments on the skin and partly to protect from scratching.

For a while bandaging went right out of fashion and was even seen as a bad thing, shutting the skin from fresh air and sunshine and restricting movement, quite apart from creating a great deal of extra work.

But over the last few years bandages impregnated with coal tar, icthammol paste and calamine have become very popular and their value appreciated.

Says Dr David Atherton, in his book *Your Child with Eczema*: 'All these bandages have a refreshing, cooling effect when applied. They can be successful in relieving irritation and also have healing properties, particularly those containing tar. Unfortunately they are quite messy to apply, and another bandage is needed to cover the wet paste bandages.

'Some people use ordinary crêpe bandages for this purpose but these are not really ideal. I find that a rather special bandage called *Coban* is best — this is elasticated and self-gripping without incorporating any adhesive.'

The bandaging process is also complicated, but Dr Atherton's book contains demonstration photographs covering the whole body from top to toe.

Parents and patients also have their own ingenious answers, as usual. Comments one mother who uses paste bandages regularly on her two children, Edward and Alice:

'As it is so messy, I keep all the old socks and use these to cover up the affected limb — often cutting out a little hole in the heel where it fits the hand so that thumb suckers can have at least one thumb for comfort!'

Avoiding Trouble

Allergy, and its connections with eczema, probably causes more confusion than any other aspect of this very complex condition. This is partly because allergy itself is a complicated subject, and partly because how much it actually triggers off eczema remains something of a mystery anyway.

As we've already seen, certain types of eczema, such as allergic contact eczema, are known to be caused by allergy. But contact eczema can also be caused by irritants which damage the sensitive surface of the skin.

Similarly, even though people with atopic eczema often also suffer from the more obviously allergic disorders of asthma and hayfever, the eczema itself is not necessarily caused by allergy. Instead, substances like feathers, dust and soap powder may be irritating and aggravating the vulnerable skin.

Nor does a reaction to a particular food necessarily have to be allergic. It may be that there is a food intolerance which acts on the inside of the body much as irritating factors act on the outside.

But even though allergy may not be the total cause of most eczema and finding certain culprits does not completely clear the rash, it may still play a significant part in some cases and is certainly worth looking into.

Allergic response

To start with, it helps to understand a little of the body's allergic mechanism. As one specialist explains, allergy is basically an exaggerated response of the immune system — which normally protects the body from attack by illnesses such as measles, sore throats and boils. But in the allergic person it can react to a whole range of things, from dust to cow's milk or pollen.

'The simplest type to explain is the asthma/hayfever allergy,' says this specialist. 'There are what are called mast cells in all the lining membranes of the body — skin, eyes, nose, respiratory tract, digestive tract. It is easiest to view these cells as small hand grenades stuck all over the inside of us, choc-a-block with chemicals, a large part of which is histamine.

'When a pollen grain hits your nose, if you have hayfever it lands on the surface of the mast cells, a message goes inside, and out pop these little chemical granules releasing the histamine.'

Allergen or antigen is the name given to a particular substance which causes allergy in a person; sensitization is the process by which this allergy comes about; and antibodies are the proteins circulating in the blood-stream which fight away invading allergen by helping the mast cells release histamine.

If a person has asthma the body's reaction to this release of chemicals will be coughing and wheezing. When someone has hayfever, the eyes and nose will stream and itch, triggering off sneezing.

The reaction of the skin is a rather more complicated process, but the lumps, bumps and redness of urticaria and hives is one result, and in certain people the reaction to all this histamine may well be eczema.

The whole process is really an inappropriate and over-dramatic response of the body to what are mostly quite harmless things, and which in the person without this particular problem would cause no reaction at all.

In his book *Diseases of Civilisation* Brain Inglis comically likens the process to an influx of tourists to a country leading to a false alarm of enemy invasion, with troops pouring out into the countryside, disrupting normal life in the process.

But as he goes on to point out, even though answers may have been found to the question of what happens when there is an allergic response, we are not much nearer to knowing *why* the body should react like this to false alarms. Many people are researching the subject and when they do come up with the answers they may also be able to shed more light on just how eczema and allergy are connected.

Taking action
In the meantime, most people with eczema and those who care for them

are finding it increasingly helpful to allow for the fact that allergy may be a factor in at any rate worsening the condition, and acting accordingly.

The only time when this may become harmful is when a whole life becomes ruled by fears of allergy or sensitivity and enemies are seen looming round every corner. To spend every hour of the day looking for possible culprits can be soul-destroying.

Apart from anything else, some people may be sensitive to so many things that it is very difficult to pin them all down. Also, the sensitivity can be to substances which are almost impossible to avoid.

But to take practical steps because observation has shown you that certain things do appear to make the eczema worse makes sense. As Dr A. W. Franklin says in his book *Allergies: Questions and Answers*, allergy or general sensitivity can be similar to having a nail in your shoe. The real treatment won't be to apply ointment to the resulting sore, but to remove the nail.

This same specialist explains how to detect signs of sensitivity or allergy. First you must watch yourself or your child over a period of time. If irritation or scratching begins, it could show a recent exposure to something triggering the rash. The reaction may not come until the next day, however, so if the skin becomes progressively worse over a period of time, the trick lies in noting details about the day before as well.

Was there any unusual or different exposure? Were strange contacts made on that day or anything unusual eaten? It will help to make a list of everything you can recall which might be a factor, including emotional upsets, exertion or overheating.

You can then check any suspicious factor by purposely exposing yourself or your child to that item and noticing if this repeatedly makes the skin and eczema flare up. Patch testing, described on page 21, may also be used to confirm reactions.

This specialist, like many others who are interested, takes it for granted that there will be help on hand if it seems likely there are allergic factors involved in the eczema. In our experience, and that of many others, it is hard to find GPs or dermatologists who are particularly convinced by allergy.

Many still pooh-pooh the idea, thinking it cranky and decidedly unnecessary to drink goat's milk or avoid additives or worry overmuch about things like dust and feathers. This may be for the sort of reasons already discussed, but the more enlightened doctors at least feel it is worth a try.

Even then, it can be difficult finding immunologists who specialize in allergy, and many allergy clinics are privately run and expensive. But some treatment is available on the NHS, and organizations like the Hyperactive Children's Support Group, Action Against Allergy and the National Society for Research into Allergy may be able to help (addresses on page 150).

Avoidance of allergens and irritants and the enforcement of a healthier diet are also the cornerstones of almost all the alternative therapies such as homoeopathy, naturopathy, acupuncture and herbalism, and this is an important first reason why many with eczema turn to them for help.

As we will see in later chapters, the practitioners treat the whole person, seeing their lives and personalities as important factors in deciding what treatment is suitable, and in a condition such as eczema this is extremely important.

Avoidance regime

But there is still a lot the patient and the family can do without a great deal of outside help, and there are certain avoidance rules to follow which have been shown to help almost all people with eczema.

Says one mother: 'The sort of precautions I stick to rigidly for my child are as follows — keep the child cool, always putting cotton next to the skin and for bedding use cotton sheets; no blankets, but instead a non-allergic continental quilt.

'Shake all bedding out of the window daily and vacuum the mattress; dust and vacuum bedroom daily but not while the child is in the room. Wash clothes in soap flakes, rinse very thoroughly and dry outside rather than in tumble drier. No pets — we just have a goldfish! Bath water should be warm with a soap substitute and a cold "hot water bottle" is helpful in summer.

'Do let the child know that his eczema is in no way catching so that he can tell his friends, and create a happy and relaxed atmosphere in the home, giving lots of cuddles and kissing as the child may feel untouchable. Above all, know that you are doing your best and have confidence in this.'

In a few words this mother puts into a nutshell some simple rules that can help keep the eczema under control and lessen the distress, emotionally as well as physically.

What to wear

Keep cool and keep comfortable — those are the two most important factors when thinking about clothes and eczema. From the tiniest baby to the oldest adult, clothing needs to be soft to the touch, absorbent and non-restrictive.

The ideal answer is all-cotton clothing, including sweaters and even coats, but many people compromise by using cotton next to the skin so that at least there is no direct contact with irritating materials such as wool or synthetic fibres.

In fact, wool and synthetics are an interesting illustration of the allergy versus irritation theory we have been discussing in this chapter. Many people used to think that because wool or nylon made the rash worse they were 'allergic' to these materials.

But modern theory is that wool is so scratchy, hot and harsh to the touch that it irritates the skin and could bring anyone out in a rash, eczema sufferer or not. Similarly, synthetics such as nylon and polyester do not allow the skin to breathe and cause over-heating and sweatiness, which again irritates the skin and causes rashes.

Some people can get away with polyester and cotton mixtures as long as the proportion of cotton is fairly high, and an acrylic mix can be a useful stand-by if it is loosely woven or knitted and feels soft. Silk is another possibility, although it is an expensive answer and may not suit everyone.

Luckily cotton yarn and clothing is much more widely available than it used to be, including colourful tights and fashionable children's outfits. Whereas when our son was young we had to search in all sorts of unlikely places such as old-fashioned haberdashery stores for cotton garments, now the most modern and trendy shops have anything from cotton multi-patterned sweaters to attractive underclothes.

You still have to keep a careful watch, however, even when clothes are sold as 'all cotton'. One mother, Dorothy Pearson, started her own cotton clothes mail order service because of the hidden dangers in many of the clothes she bought her 4-year-old daughter.

'I spent a long time tracking down garments, particularly those worn next to the skin, such as night clothes, tights and underwear,' she explains. 'I would triumphantly take home some cotton knee-socks, but when Hannah wore them she would come out in a rash behind her knees because of elastic at the top of the socks.

'Or little cotton vests would leave scarlet weals around neckline and arms where the 'all-cotton' garment had been trimmed with nylon lace or stitched with nylon thread. I eventually found Swedish cotton tights, but they were £6.50 a pair. I got so tired searching that I decided to so something about it myself.'

Her designs have no nylon or elastic in trimmings, underwear has soft bound edges and, for babies, envelope necks, and children's outfits often have built-in feet and mittens to minimize scratching, especially at night.

The address of Dorothy's firm *Cotton On* is listed at the back of this book, but for an update on information you can always contact the National Eczema Society who also have useful leaflets on the subject, including one especially about children's clothes.

Remember it can be the dressing or dye in new clothes that causes irritation, so it is a good idea to wash and rinse before wearing. One woman found her contact eczema was caused by the dye in nylon stockings, so from then on she bought undyed tights and coloured them herself with *Dylon*.

So, check what you wear from top to bottom — literally! One recent study found that both young men and women were developing rashes around the tops of their legs and on their behinds because of tight denim jeans. So keep clothes as loose as possible, particularly round the crutch and underarms.

Others find that shoes can cause problems, from the synthetic material to the dyes used in the leather. One adult with eczema, Eileen Horan, says that shoes lined with foam are very bad for her and she avoids them at all costs. She even removes the small strips of foam used under the inner sole and substitutes cotton wool instead.

'Other shoes have nylon lining, and this, too, isn't good,' Eileen writes. 'Unlined leather shoes are best. In winter I avoid slippers with synthetic linings (many have foam) and I always wear leather moccasins. In summer I wear sandals as much as possible, as I have found that the cooler my feet are, the better it is for the eczema.'

Sweet dreams

Many eczema sufferers appear to have most discomfort at night, which is probably due to a mixture of overheating, the wrong sort of bedding and perhaps a build-up of tension because of the subsequent itchiness and need to scratch.

To lessen the problems the number one rule again is to go for coolness and comfort, and there are many practical steps you can take to alleviate the difficulties. First, loose pyjamas and nightdresses in cotton for adults or all-in-one cotton sleepsuits for babies and young children are the best sort of nightwear.

Ideally, sheets should be all cotton, but for some a mixture of polyester and cotton is suitable. This also cuts down on washing problems, as sheets need to be washed regularly and there is often the added staining from blood and sticky ointments. Cotton flannelette sheets are a cuddly alternative but they are more of a chore to wash and dry, and can cause overheating in bed.

If blankets are used, they should be the cotton cellular type popular in hospitals, and these are particularly suitable for young babies.

However, most adults with eczema find that duvets or continental quilts, cotton-covered and with a non-allergic synthetic filling, are best. For summer, a thin version called a duvette may be even more suitable — and all duvets have the advantage that they can be washed or cleaned easily.

Pillows should also have a synthetic filling and cotton covers. Not only are feathers an irritant in themselves, they are a natural dust trap and difficult to keep clean. The same feather-free rule applies to mattresses, which should be made from synthetic materials and never be filled with kapok, disintegrating cotton, straw or horsehair.

Old, mouldy mattresses which may have been damaged by bed-wetting should be replaced, as they can be a prime source of irritation and even allergy. Ideally, the mattress should also be encased in a fitted plastic cover since this is an added protection from irritation and also makes the mattress easier to clean.

Down with dust

The general aim should be to keep the whole bedroom as sterile and dust-free as possible, with vinyl covering on the floor, perhaps adding a few rugs for comfort. Blinds at the window are less of a dust trap than curtains, and furniture and ornaments should be easy-to-clean.

The reason for all this care is because tests have shown that dust, and the dust mite which lives off it, can be a prime source of allergy and irritation. There is also the fact, as already mentioned, that dust mites like eating dried skin flakes, and find the bed and room of the eczema sufferer a very happy hunting ground for hearty meals.

So it is sensible to shake out bedding and rugs and vacuum mattress and bedroom daily, perhaps using one of the extra powerful models now on the market. Then, once a week, damp dust the room and the mattress cover, also washing bedding at regular intervals.

There can be a danger of becoming over-worried and obsessive about dust and this should be guarded against. The normal, comfortable home will obviously have a certain amount of dust about, but if you can at least keep it to a minimum and make a particular effort in the bedroom, this could pay dividends.

An adult patient has found that desensitizing injections have helped his confirmed allergy to dust and dust mites and led to what he describes as a miraculous improvement.

'I was previously a semi-invalid, but the condition is now only a fraction as bad and is still improving,' he says. 'The rash was so severe that I gave up work eighteen months ago, but now I hope to be able to get a job again.'

It is also possible now to kill the dust mite off at source. A product called *Tymasil* can be sprayed onto the mattress once a week, destroying the mould which forms on skin scales and other household debris contained in dust, and therefore denying the mite its staple diet.

Caution with cosmetics

Cosmetics and toiletries can cause problems but, yet again, this is not necessarily because of allergy but because the product contains ingredients which irritate an already sensitive skin.

Mostly, it is a question of trial and error to find out which cream, lipstick or talcum powder is suitable and which is not, although some are more regular offenders than others. For instance, deodorants, sunscreening products, depilatories, hair dyes and aftershave can all act as irritants as well as an allergen causing contact eczema.

Also, it is often just one ingredient in the product that is causing the trouble — for instance perfume, lanolin, preservative or colouring. That is why some people find hypoallergenic cosmetics and toiletries helpful, because these are specially made with many of the more common allergens and irritants left out.

In one brand over sixty ingredients often used in cosmetic formulation have been blacklisted. These include natural perfume oils, corn starch, crude lanolin, certain resins, indelible dyes, orris root, cocoa butter, henna and herb compounds. The ranges also undergo laboratory and dermatological tests before reaching the shop counter.

Another advantage of these products is that they often list ingredients on the package or with an accompanying leaflet, and if you have discovered you are sensitive to any particular substance it is easier to avoid it.

Wash day blues

Other common irritants to be avoided are some of the modern laundry products which lure us with their claims to whiter whites and instant spotlessness. Considering the sort of washing load that some eczema patients and their families have, it isn't surprising we are tempted!

But, in the main, it is far safer to use the milder soap flakes and soap-based powders for handwashing and top-loading automatics and twin tubs, and the low-lather detergent powders and liquids for front loading automatic machines.

Because the biological and low-temperature powders and liquids have to contain enzymes and other irritant ingredients to work their magic on stains and dirt, these are difficult to rinse out completely and can leave a residue on the washing which affects the skin.

This all came to a head when one leading manufacturer abandoned its original mild washing powder and introduced a 'new system' biological product which brought hundreds of people out in a rash and aggravated the atopic eczema of many more. As a result of public and press outcry, the manufacturers returned their original product to the shop shelves.

Experiment with powders and liquids to find one that is suitable, but it's best to avoid fabric conditioners and strong perfumes, particularly when washing a baby's nappies, and whatever the product, very thorough rinsing is necessary to remove every trace of the washing product used.

Up to the individual

These, then, are the basic avoidance measures that seem to help most eczema sufferers. The rest tends to be up to the individual, as reactions will vary from one person to another.

Allergies or sensitivity to grasses, pollen, tree spores and moulds are difficult to avoid and could even involve a move to a different part of the country. Reaction to heat and cold, soft and hard water, wet or dry climate, may all play a part in eczema. But more about these factors in Chapter 13, 'Out in the World'.

Desensitization by injection has already been mentioned, but a method growing in popularity is enzyme potentated desensitization. Once strong allergies have been detected, 'cocktails' containing a dilution of the offending substances are made up and administered in the form of drops, usually placed under the tongue, over a period of time.

According to one woman with eczema who was in the middle of a course of treatment when I talked to her, grasses, pollens, various foods and many other allergens are suitable for the cocktails. The body builds up a defence, and if treatment is successful it should be possible to eat or do whatever you wish, without any ill effects.

Sometimes emotions are a deciding factor in what we can live with and what we must avoid. For instance, many eczema sufferers are sensitive to animals and react to their hairs and dander and sometimes saliva. But the affection and comfort gained from having a beloved pet has to be weighed against the possible physical dangers.

Says one animal lover: 'When my cat died I was strongly advised not to have another. For over a year my asthma was worse and my hands were raw with eczema. We could stand it no longer without an animal so we got two Tibetian spaniels.

'I am as well as I have ever been and any day I am going to get a kitten for my dogs as they love cats as we do. The psychological harm done by longing for or missing an animal is far worse than the slight effect they *may* have on you.'

Food is another area of dilemma. My son loves beefburgers and milk, but these could be the very reason his eczema continues. Yet so far I have been unsuccessful in persuading him to give them up as he sees this as yet another trial on top of all the others caused by eczema.

So, for more about how to cope with diet, read on.

Finding Out About Food

For many people, a change in diet is the crucial factor in the successful control of eczema. Certainly it is the key to most of the alternative methods explored in this book, the underlying philosophy being 'you are what you eat'.

The use of creams and ointments and even the avoidance of substances like feathers and dust, is approaching the problem from the outside of the body and may simply be a way of suppressing the symptoms.

But paying attention to the food we eat and planning a careful diet can get to the root of the problem. In the case of eczema, the symptoms are being attacked from the inside with the hope of finding first the cause, and then perhaps the cure.

On the face of it this seems a simple and obvious approach and, of course, there is nothing very new about it. For years people have believed that skin disorders are an outside sign of something wrong inside, whether this was acne caused by fatty foods or boils by 'bad blood'.

But the reality is a lot more complicated, and although many people do find that diet affects their eczema, there are no hard and fast rules and reactions vary a great deal from person to person.

So, the same page of *Exchange* carries letters from two mothers, one of whom tried goat's instead of cow's milk and found that within two days there was a dramatic improvement in her daugher's eczema. The other found just the opposite.

Says the first mother: 'We have unbroken nights and a happy child. I don't pretend to understand what is going on or why this should happen — I only know without any doubt that it has.'

Says the second mother: 'I tried goat's milk, sure that it would cure him because everyone, including my GP and my dermatologist, said it was beneficial. But I was in the depths of despair when the baby was terribly sick every day, and was losing weight.'

This mother eventually found that a type of soya milk was the answer and her baby's skin has improved so much on this vegetable milk that neighbours call in especially to see him 'no longer red and weeping all over.'

But a third mother reports that her son reacts to all beans, including soya. 'His eczema deteriorated when he began school dinners, and then we realized that the school serves soya protein instead of meat. So a vegetarian diet doesn't seem to be the answer for us,' she concludes.

Adult reactions

This diversity of reactions and attitudes to diet is even more pronounced when it comes to adults. One lady who had suffered from severe eczema for twenty-eight years switched from cow's milk to goat's milk and reports:

'It was the changing point of my life. From the first carton the improvement was dramatic — nobody would believe it — I was a different person. When I look back on my many years of trying to keep my sanity while struggling with rubber gloves, ointments and every so-called remedy under the sun, I only regret that no doctor ever put me on a diet. Yet it's so simple.'

But on the very next page of *Exchange* another adult patient writes: 'It would appear that some people are certain that all eczema is caused by food allergies and if you are not aware of any in your particular case then you are virtually incompetent. But I have no evidence that I am affected by certain foods.'

I do not quote these letters to undermine the good effects that changes in diet can have, and which are borne out by the hundreds of positive letters which pour into the National Eczema Society and its magazine. But they do illustrate the important point that everyone is different and that what helps one won't necessarily help another — and some, in fact, may not be helped at all.

This proved to be the case when our son was younger. We tried many diets when he was a child, including goat's milk, vegan and non-wheat, and sometimes he did show signs of improvement for a while. Then back would come the symptoms with a vengeance, and there would be a feeling of failure all round.

Being aware that diet may not help can save parents and patients from guilt and self-recrimination if things don't work, and also from getting caught on an obsessive tread-mill of more and more stringent dieting until the poor person can hardly eat anything at all.

Apart from being stressful and depressing, this can also be very dangerous, as the diet may be lacking in essential nutrients. Far from improving the eczema it may actually cause other illnesses and dramatic loss of weight.

So it is important to seek advice and guidance from experts. Many hospitals now have dieticians who can give help, and practitioners of the various alternative therapies also study diet and use this as part of their treatments.

Food intolerance

So far I have purposefully tried to avoid the use of the words 'food allergy'. This is because, just as outside agents act as an irritant, causing or aggravating eczema in different ways, so can inside agents such as food. But this does not necessarily indicate allergy in the true sense of the word.

Explains Dr David Atherton: 'Parents frequently notice that tomatoes make the area round a child's mouth red, and other foods which tend to do this are oranges and *Marmite*. Such children may be truly allergic to these foods, but the redness is more often simply a consequence of direct irritation due to acidity of tomatoes and oranges, or the saltiness of the *Marmite*.

'In some children certain foods may cause a more intense reaction than just redness when they come into direct contact with the skin. Most characteristically this will take the form of weals at the site of the contact, usually on the face, but often on the fingers and hands as well. This reaction is known in medical language as contact urticaria.'

Dr Atherton points out that this may be a genuine allergy, but it is not the same as the eczema and the food may cause no problem at all when swallowed. On the other hand it may have an effect, and in some cases may even cause eczema.

Because of these differences in the ways that food can affect the skin and the eczema, many doctors prefer the term 'food intolerance', as this covers the sort of sensitivity described here as well as other more chemical reactions and clear-cut allergies.

Another vital factor to bear in mind is that, even if eczema cannot all be put down to nervous causes, anxiety or general debility can play a part in food intolerance or allergy.

Explains Valerie Hall, a young woman who has had eczema since childhood: 'Having been told by all the experts that food was definitely not a factor in eczema, I was sceptical. Still, I got a copy of *Not All in the Mind* by Richard Mackarness and there I found a paragraph that started my cure.

Dr Mackarness said that most people assume that the emotion causes the allergy, whereas he believes that the emotion causes only an exhaustion of protective hormones, thus lowering the defences against allergy to a substance that otherwise might not cause any trouble.

'Whether you actually develop symptoms will depend on the state of your adaptive defences at the time. You are more likely to react if you have been battling with a cold, or a broken love affair, or been at loggerheads with a loved one, than if you are in robust health, happy and settled.'

Eventually Valerie found that tea, cheese, ham, chicken, pork and chocolate were the main offenders in her diet and, having removed them, within a few weeks her skin was completely back to normal.

Breast-feeding

Many in the medical profession are still very sceptical about food intolerance as a cause of eczema, and are often happier to hand over the latest steroid preparation than recommend a dietician or a diet sheet.

This seems a pity since, as long as dieting is done carefully and with some supervision, it should do no harm and may do a great deal of good. Even if diet makes no difference, experimenting removes the nagging uncertainty that food may be the source of the eczema.

The lack of interest on the part of some doctors is because they feel there is not enough medical evidence to prove the worth of dieting in the treatment of eczema. But recent studies by Dr Atherton and other leading specialists has shown that, in a proportion of babies and children, allergy avoidance of all sorts can make a great deal of difference.

For instance, a study at the Institute of Child Health observed the results when 'at risk' babies (whose parents had eczema and therefore stood a high chance of developing the condition) were kept off cow's milk and preferably breast-fed for the first months of life.

As far as possible the babies were also kept away from other possible irritants and allergens such as feathers, dust, woollen clothing and so on, so that a fair assessment of their progress could be made.

The results were compared with a group where such an avoidance regime was not kept, and showed that the avoidance babies were less likely to develop eczema than otherwise. This continued to be true even when being introduced to solid foods, but these were chosen with care and reactions watched all the time.

Studies since have shown that it is also important what a mother herself eats while she is breast-feeding, and if possible she should avoid the more obvious allergy-provoking foods such as eggs and cow's milk.

On the other hand, a nursing mother needs a highly nutritious diet and if she cuts out these foods from her daily diet, then she should have an alternative source of protein in the form of extra meat and calcium tablets, and should also consult a dietician or some other expert.

There are some who believe that it is the breast-milk itself and not the avoidance of cow's milk that is so beneficial for the eczema and one specialist has been working on a study to treat older children and even adults with human breast milk expressed by nursing mothers.

This milk has been used mostly for children with allergic rhinitis, in the form of nose drops, but the specialist has also given it orally to four children with atopic eczema. One improved remarkably, and another responded to the milk applied to the skin in the form of a cream.

There is one organization, Foresight, which campaigns for improved preconceptual care, believing that if mothers and fathers both ate a more nutritional diet and kept their bodies fit, then pregnancy and babies would be healthier.

This organization, like many others, is particularly worried by the refined and convenience foods which have become a regular part of modern eating, and believes that these deplete the body of essential vitamins, and trace minerals such as zinc.

Certainly some recent research has shown a steep rise in the number of people suffering from eczema in the last 15 years or so, and this, it is suggested, is a result of additives in food and general pollution with chemicals and pesticides. The doctors involved feel a great deal more research is needed into this aspect.

Tracing the culprits

Meanwhile individuals can carry out their own investigations into what does and doesn't suit them. Because babies are usually on such a simple diet, i.e. mother's or bottled milk, it is simpler to assess any food intolerance they may have.

If a baby is regularly sick or doubled up with colic or breaks out in a rash, then there are not many foods you can suspect. Even as babies grow and are weaned, the number of solids suitable are limited, and it is therefore easier to watch for reactions.

But as he or she gets older the number and types of foods and food ingredients grows, too, and finding the culprits (if there are any) becomes a more complicated business. With adults the search becomes even more involved because there are yet more possibilities, including alcohol, rich and spicy foods, tea and coffee.

Just as with outside irritants or allergens such as dust, feathers and straw, the first step is observation. If every time a certain food is eaten the rash becomes worse, or there is some other bodily change such as flushing, irritation or swelling, there is obvious reason for suspicion.

Sometimes the reaction can be so extreme, as in *oedema*, that there is swelling of the tissues inside the body, such as the throat, which causes choking and even suffocation. When this happens a food must obviously be avoided at all costs.

Along with observation, skin tests can also be a helpful pointer. A small amount of a suspected food or other substance is held against the skin or pricked into it and then left covered for forty-eight hours. If redness or irritation develops, there could be allergy.

But on its own this is not a reliable method since a rash may not mean there is allergy or even intolerance. On the other hand a test may confirm very strong suspicions based on other evidence.

Natural detections

Other methods of detection used particularly in the field of natural medicine are hair analysis through radionics, and dowsing, when a pendulum is swung over the body to confirm or deny allergies (more about this in Chapter 7). Some use the pulse method, based on the principle that when the body reacts unfavourably to food, the pulse rate will go up.

Explains one young patient: 'I have cured myself of eczema which I have suffered since the age of two months by cutting out foods to which I found I was allergic. I found these foods by this simple pulse test:

1. Check pulse after relaxing for two minutes.
2. Eat the food to be tested.
3. Check pulse while still resting at intervals of 10, 20, 40 and 60 minutes.

'If, on these counts, the pulse should rise by more than 10 beats per minute, it is likely that one is allergic to the food. It should then be avoided in all its forms. In my case (and I stress that other sufferers may be different) the foods are milk, eggs, butter, cheese, bacon, grapefruit juice and white beet sugar.'

Other adults have tried a short fast, although this method should not be used with children, or if an adult is generally unwell or becomes ill during the fast. But one adult fasted with a successful outcome under the guidance of a private allergy clinic.

'The fast was relatively easy,' she writes. 'All I was allowed was water, and bottled at that. But I managed to look after my two pre-school and two school-age children. The only time I felt a bit weak was when we went into the local supermarket to do the weekend shopping.

'After a week's fasting my skin cleared completely from head to toe. I had been warned I might get withdrawal symptoms and in fact for the first few days my skin seemed to get worse. But then it started to improve, not just the rash but all the thick, hard flaky skin got better, too.

'I have been told to stop using all ointments and medicines. This I thought would be impossible but I was able to comply. All I used during the fast and since was Boots' E45 emollient cream which I find invaluable, plus an emollient in the bath.

'After this I had to test reintroduction of foods by the pulse method and am now on a wheatless and dairyless diet. The eczema comes back if I stray from my straight and narrow eating habits, and adapting to a new way of eating is strange and not always easy. But the results are well worth it.'

Elimination diets

By far the most common method for testing food intolerance in children and adults is the exclusion or elimination diet. By this method you either cut from your daily intake the foods you personally suspect are damaging, or the ones that are most commonly thought to affect eczema — for instance, cow's milk, eggs, gluten and wheat, nuts, fish and additives such as preservatives and colourings.

The difficulty with this type of diet is that it isn't just a single food that must be eliminated, but other foods that contain it. So if the diet is cow's milk-free it's no good simply doing away with the daily pinta. Cheese, butter, yogurt, biscuits, bread and anything else containing cow's milk or its constituents must be eliminated, too.

Similarly, when excluding additives and colourings, these will be found in almost every manufactured food on the shelves of supermarket and stores. Even some medicines include yellow colouring, such as antihistamine syrups prescribed for eczema, so ingredients and labels must be checked carefully.

At Great Ormond Street Hospital the specialists often put children on an egg- and milk-free diet to avoid chicken at the same time, because some of the proteins in chicken and egg are identical.

Says Dr David Atherton, in a diet leaflet especially for children: 'If an egg- and milk-free diet is going to help it will usually do so within four or six weeks. The full benefit may not be seen if the diet is abandoned too early. If it does prove helpful, the diet should ideally be maintained unchanged for about a year, and the dietician should check on the nutritional adequacy of the diet at least once during this time.

'At the end of the year you will need to find out whether these foods can now be eaten without problems. This is best done by trying eliminated foods again, one by one. Ideally a full week should be set aside for each item. If this were milk, for example, a teaspoon only should be given on the first day if there is any reason to believe that an allergy may be intense.

'If not, you can give a full glass of milk on the first day. If no adverse effects are apparent following this first dose, give between half and a full pint on each of the next six days. If at any time the eczema becomes worse again, stop the reintroduction, although if you feel there may be another explanation for the deterioration, you could try again later.'

On the other hand, if the reintroduction shows that there is a definite intolerance to a particular food or to several foods, the diet should continue.

Wider exclusion

If there are no initial clues as to which foods might be causing problems, then a wider exclusion diet may be necessary. This could cut out several groups of foods, including eggs, cow's milk, wheat and even coffee.

The book *The Allergy Diet* written by doctors and a dietician at Addenbrooke's Hospital in Cambridge explains clearly and in great detail how to follow such a diet safely and successfully, listing the foods to avoid and the foods that are safe.

Basically the authors suggest that the exclusion diet should be kept to strictly for two weeks, with an accurate diary kept of which foods are eaten and what symptoms, if any, occur. This will also help pinpoint unusual food sensitivity not normally suspected.

The book also gives a list for reintroducing foods in a recommended order, starting with tap water and tomatoes, and finishing with wheat, nuts and preservatives. Again, reactions must be carefully noted and the food withdrawn if there are obvious signs of the eczema becoming worse.

A rotation diet follows much the same principle, except that certain groups of foods are eaten on certain days for a number of weeks so they come round once every four to seven days.

Out of all this effort may come the confirmation that food intolerance plays little part in the eczema. But if improvements are great enough, then a long-term diet will be worth the effort.

6.

Diets in Action

Embarking on a diet once food intolerance is suspected or has been definitely confirmed is an exciting challenge and gives the rewarding feeling you are doing something positive about the eczema.

On the other hand dieting can be a difficult and time-consuming occupation, needing a great deal of determination and perseverance. This is particularly so when the diet must be long-term, lacking some of the pioneering feel of elimination experiments.

Knowing that from now on you can't drink alcohol or eat wheat bread or have sugar in your tea can make you want those 'forbidden fruits' even more. Rather like the slimmer craving cakes or fudge, the desire to have an occasional fling can become overwhelming.

Interestingly, dietary experts have noticed that it is often the best-loved foods that may be causing the problems. The toddler who drinks pints of milk may, in fact, be wanting the very food that is worst for him or her.

So the important basic rule for any diet, whichever foods are being excluded, is to settle into a fairly strict routine which keeps temptation at bay as far as possible. This may mean some thorough research initially, plus planning of menu and food cupboard so that the right foods are at hand when needed.

Writes one mother: 'Sitting in the kitchen late one evening with the list of to-have and have-nots on my lap, the diet looked distinctly daunting. To provide meals for a family of five which were not only milk and egg-free, but fish, beef and chicken-free too meant some careful thinking and research.

'We had decided that the only sensible course was to try the diet without compromises, and during that time all the family must eat the same food. My husband and I went through the larder checking all the labels and the 'outs' were stowed away in the large box well out of reach and sight of the family.

'The following morning was spent visiting various food stores and checking over their labels for ingredients before purchase. Naturally this took a little time at first, but one quickly got used to it.

'There were three more things to do before countdown — enlist the help of the school staff over lunches; make sure I had a good exercise book to keep a record of all the food and drink taken with reactions and skin changes; and, finally, to tell our dear son what was in store for him!'

Letting school and friends know what is happening is a very important part of successful dieting. To stick to the rules at home and then find that all the wrong foods are being offered outside can defeat the whole object.

In her book of milk-, egg- and additive-free recipes called *What Can I Give Him Today?* Diana Wells suggests badges saying 'I am on a milk-free diet' or 'Please don't give me eggs' for children, particularly the really young who wouldn't be able to explain the situation.

There are many helpful books now available written by cookery and dietary experts who can advise on the ins and outs of dieting in great detail. Rita Greer, for instance, has written books on gluten-free, wheat-free, milk-free and egg-free cooking.

Her advice is not to fly into a panic, but instead to direct energy into getting organized in the kitchen in order to cope with the new situation on the domestic front. Included in her suggestions is the point that, when an allergy or food intolerance is very marked, it may be necessary to use separate cooking utensils.

'Scrupulous cleanliness is essential to avoid contamination, with extra care during the washing up,' she says. 'Egg white has a very strong tendency to attach itself to utensils, baking sheet, etc. Avoid using the same spoon to stir a non-milk drink when everyone else is having a drinking containing milk. This kind of attitude should not be considered fussy — merely careful.'

Another point to remember when planning a diet is that it is not always necessary to cut a type of food out completely, but simply to substitute it with something similar but more suitable — carob powder instead of chocolate, for example, or soya instead of wheat flour.

And don't forget label and ingredient checking. On the next pages some of the most common diets used to control eczema are listed, and in every case it will be necessary not just to eliminate the food itself but other products which contain it.

For more detailed advice you can refer to the organizations and books listed in the last section of this book, and also see a dietician if possible.

A diet will do no good at all if it creates other deficiencies in the body, and it is essential that there should be a balanced intake of all the necessary proteins, fats, carbohydrate, fibre, vitamins and minerals.

Diet for a baby

As mentioned in the last chapter, some of the clearest evidence of food intolerance contributing to eczema has come from studies on new-born and young babies. If breast-fed, or at any rate kept well away from cow's milk, they appear to stand less chance of developing eczema.

One specialist who had made a detailed study of the subject goes so far as to wonder why we regard cow's milk as a useful foodstuff at all. No other mammal on earth, he says, takes milk after it has been weaned from its mother's breast or drinks the milk of another species.

'That cow's milk is "full of goodness" has an emotive appeal, but it is true only for new born calves, and even then only provided they have received their colustrum,' the specialist adds. 'For humans it is nutritionally unsatisfactory and inferior to almost any other source of protein, carbohydrate, fat and mineral.'

Not everyone would agree with this, but certainly most mothers nowadays prefer not to resort to bottle feeds and supplementaries, at least until they have given breast-feeding a chance. Even if breast-feeding is not successful, there are nutritious soya milks which can be used in a bottle instead.

Jill Weigal had suffered from eczema on her hands all her life and when her baby was born she decided to take all the avoidance action she could, breast-feeding Catherine for nine months and not allowing any supplementary bottles when she was first born.

'The first meal I introduced solids into was the 2 p.m. feed when, after breast-feeding, Catherine was given a little raw fresh fruit, starting with really ripe, sweet apples cut in half and then scraped gently across the surface so that she had a little pulp.

'After a fortnight I introduced a tiny amount of cereal — not bought cereal, all of which contains sugar and skimmed milk, but health food rolled oats ground to a fine powder and then poached over hot water, with water added. And so we have continued, and she still starts all her meals with raw fruit, fresh and in season, such as pears, grapes and peaches.

'After six months she had cow's milk and cottage cheese and homemade wholemeal bread and yogurt. So far her skin is clear, bless her, and long may it continue to be so.'

Useful advice also comes from Dr David Atherton who recommends that introduction of solid foods should start no earlier than the fourth month and no later than the seventh. He suggests the fifth month as the ideal time, but thinks that breast-feeding should continue until the end of the first year, topping up with soya milk if necessary.

'Introduce vegetables and fruits first of all,' he suggests. 'Suitable vegetables include potatoes, lentils, peas, beans, cabbage, broccoli, brussel sprouts, cauliflower, carrots, swedes or turnips. These should be boiled carefully as over-cooking destroys much of their nutritional value, and then sieved or mashed.

'A little milk-free margarine e.g., *Tomor*, can be added for its softening effect. Potato should be preferred to cereal at this stage as a source of carbohydrate and it is a good idea to mix boiled, mashed potato with other vegetables. Introduce some minced meat after a further week or two. Turkey or lamb are a good choice as there is no overlap with egg and cow's milk, though in practice there is little risk with chicken and beef.'

After another week or two he suggests the introduction of cereals, starting with rice. Gradually expand the range of solids one at a time, but watching for any reactions. Egg, however, should be left until the baby is at least two years old if there is any reason to think he or she might be at risk of developing eczema.

Cow's milk-free

As a baby grows, many people think immediately of a goat's milk diet as an alternative to cow's milk. Rather like breast milk for young babies, they see the goat's milk as a cure in itself as if it contains some magical property. Instead it is more likely the removal of cow's milk from the diet and the use of goat's milk as a substitute that is actually doing the trick.

However, it is believed by many that goat's milk is more easily digested than cow's milk and therefore more suitable for human consumption. Apparently, the fat and protein are present in the milk in a more finely-divided state, and also have a mild laxative effect and higher content of Vitamin B_1.

But it won't do any good simply drinking a pint of goat's milk a day and carrying on eating as usual. It is necessary at the same time to plan a very careful diet looking on labels not just for milk as an ingredient, but also whey, curd and casein.

Explains one goat breeder who has supplied her goats' milk to babies, children and adults with eczema: 'While goat's milk is taken as a substitue for cow's milk all other cow's milk products should be stopped i.e., cow's butter, cream, cheese, custards, etc., and foods containing cow's milk such as chocolate, cakes, ice cream and yogurt.'

Writes a mother from Cheshire, whose daughter's eczema has been much improved on a goat's milk diet: 'A child needn't feel too deprived of goodies when he is on a diet, though I have to say I have a freezer which I find invaluable.

'I batch bake scones, small iced cakes, jam tarts, biscuits, fruit pies and gingerbread men, using my normal recipes but substituting *Tomor* kosher margarine for butter and goat's milk for cow's milk.

'You can also make cottage cheese from goat's milk and in our local health food shop I found kosher gelatine-free table jellies and also a vegetable pâté which is excellent for sandwich spreads. Sweets are a problem, but you can give apples, crisps, raisins and sultanas instead.'

One word of warning — though most goat breeders nowadays have a very high standard of milk production, there are no rules and regulations laid down for pasteurization. It is therefore best, unless you know the supplier well, to boil the milk before use, especially when it is used in a young child's diet.

It is even possible now to use sheep's or ewe's milk as a substitute for cow's and this can be made into yogurt and cheese. The British Sheep Dairying Association and the British Goat Society (addresses in the final section of this book) can give details of suppliers.

Another widely-used substitute for cow's milk is soya milk made from the soya bean. Soya is highly nutritious and many of the manufactured milks also contain added vitamins and supplements. For suggestions, see the up-to-date list in the NES diet leaflet.

Egg-free

Along with milk, eggs are another very frequent source of food intolerance. Some people are so sensitive to them that they can react to the minutest quantity and may also be unable to eat chicken.

Like milk, eggs will be found in a wide number of manufactured and shop-bought foods so that, when shopping, labels and wrappers must be checked carefully, remembering that it may be the constituents of eggs such as white (albumen), yolk or lecithin which may be mentioned.

Eggs provide protein, fat, calcium, iron and vitamins in our diet, but quite apart from their nutritional qualities are valued for their clever cooking abilities, magically making cakes and meringues rise, and rissoles and potato cakes hold together.

There are substitute products which can take over these raising and binding qualities, or baking powder can be used — replacing each egg with two teaspoons of baking powder. These do not replace the nutritional value of eggs, however, and the diet will have to be adjusted accordingly, for instance adding more meat and fish if this is allowed.

Many milk-free diets are also egg-free, as people with one sensitivity also seem to have the other. Though eliminating both may appear a mammoth task, home-cooking and plenty of good recipe books can provide a surprisingly varied diet.

One mother of a child whose diet excludes not only eggs and all cow products, but also pork, chocolate and fish, includes among her suggestions for a daily menu:

'For breakfast you can have porridge oats with water, sugar and pineapple; toasted banana sandwiches; bread and jam; cornflakes and orange juice.

'At lunch and supper always have soups, preferably home-made so that you can control the ingredients. Mushrooms on toast are tasty and so is mince with fried onions added, bound with bread crumbs and baked in a roll using puff pastry. Chicken in all its forms, turkey or veal schnitzels, risottos, spaghetti using tomato sauce as a topping, lamb chops.

'For desserts I do treacle tart, baked apples, apple dumplings and anything with pastry — you do not need an egg for good pastry. Try making cream horns using puff pastry and fill with jam and a butter cream substituting *Tomor* margarine. Custard is acceptable using water instead of milk.'

Wheat-free

Wheat is another food high on the list of regular offenders, though it often seems to get overlooked as far as eczema goes. But wheat allergy is common enough to make it a possibility and a diet worth trying.

In some people, for instance those with coeliac disease, it is the gluten content of wheat grains and also of rye, barley and oats that causes the problem and gluten-free flours can be used as a substitute in cooking.

Others, who may have an intolerance to wheat as a whole, can use substitutes such as buckwheat, millet, potato flour, rye, rice and soya flour. All of these, particularly the gluten-free products, lack the properties which make light, fluffy bread but with care it is possible to cook an acceptable imitation.

I well remember the hours I used to spend making batter-based bread when our son was on first a gluten-free, then a wheat-free diet, and the disappointing results which looked rather like an unrisen Yorkshire pudding! But there are now much better substitute flours, and you can also buy types of wheat-free bread, such as rye.

However, wheat can be a difficult ingredient to avoid, and labels should be studied carefully. Gravy powder, tinned baked beans, cocoa, curry powder and even pickles can contain wheat. Baking powder and starch also have to be avoided, and wheat flour is often added to ground white pepper.

Cross contamination can also be a problem. Wheat, rye, barley, oats and rice are traditionally stored, milled and packed in the same factories and the wheat dust can affect other cereals. So before buying check that alternative cereals are guaranteed wheat-free.

In the home, too, wheat-free ingredients and cooking utensils should be stored separately, and crumbs from both kinds of bread can accumulate at the bottom of toaster or grill.

Although this may all seem very complicated, once you have stocked the food cupboard with the right products, including wheat-free cereals and drinks, and mastered the basics of wheat-free bread and cakes, much of the family's ordinary meals including meat, vegetable and fruit dishes will make a suitable menu.

Additive-free

As we've already seen, eczema appears to have become more widespread in recent years, and certain studies have put this down to the increasing uses of additives such as colourings, flavourings and presevatives in our foods.

Some of these additives are natural, necessary or harmless. But others are not necessary in that they are used to artificially enhance the appearance or taste of foods, and are also thought to be damaging to health.

Tinned peas are dyed green to make them look fresh, kippers are dyed yellow to make them more appetizing and orange squash is made to look even more orange than a real orange. Even butter is often coloured, and chickens are fed dyes to make egg yolks a deeper shade of gold.

One of the worst culprits appears to be tartrazine (E102), nick-named 'the yellow peril', which is an orange/yellow dye used to colour foods, soft drinks and drugs, including medicine syrups and the coating on capsules and tablets.

At first it was thought only to aggravate conditions such as urticaria, asthma and hyperactivity in children. But when the Hyperactive Children's Support Group started using additive-free diets they found that children with eczema were improving, too.

Now many parents of children with eczema and adult patients are experimenting with a diet which cuts out all additives, often with success. Writes Vicki Jones, mother of a little girl who had suffered from atopic eczema and urticaria since ten months old:

'Since both disappeared during occasional bouts of illness when she was unable to eat or drink, we always suspected dietary irritants. We are vegetarians and fairly food-conscious, so I always noticed that her eczema worsened after parties or meals at friends' houses where she ate more "kid's food" than she does at home.

'I was alerted to an article on allergy and food colouring and investigated her blackcurrant "health" drink. She stopped having it and her urticaria disappeared immediately, her sores began to heal on arms and legs, she was more temperate in her moods and slept much better.'

Another mother Barbara Newton writes: 'We discovered that tartrazine was causing our son's eczema and since avoiding this his asthma has also improved. We avoid all green, yellow and orange foods, drinks and sweets when colouring has been added (especially orange squash), and even yellow breadcrumbs as on fish fingers.'

The Feingold Diet

The Hyperactive Children's Support Group recommend the Feingold Diet as a way of testing for additive allergy. Under this diet, two groups of food are eliminated.

Group 1 includes all food and drinks containing the following additives, synthetic colouring and flavouring: monosodium glutomate; sodium glutomate; nitrates; sodium benzoate; butylated hydroxyanisole (BHA) and butylated hydroxytoluene (BHT); and benzoic acid.

Group 2 covers fruits, nuts and vegetables containing natural salicyclate to which some children can be sensitive. These include almonds, apples, apricots, peaches, plums, prunes, oranges, tomatoes, tangerines, cucumber, blackberries, strawberries, raspberries, gooseberries, cherries, currants, grapes and raisins.

These must be avoided for four to six weeks in any form — fresh, frozen, tinned, dried, as juice or as an ingredient of prepared foods. Later they can be reintroduced one at a time and if there is no worsening of the eczema or other symptoms, they can be added to the daily diet again.

The Hyperactive Children's Support Group produce a very helpful booklet listing safe foods and ideas for meals, plus recipes. All additives are now being given 'E' numbers for easier identification on labelling, and there is a list of references at the end of this book.

And by the way, it is not only manufactured foods that must be watched for additives. Janet Norris, who had suffered from eczema for many years and found she was sensitive to tartrazine, also discovered there were other hidden additives in the food we eat.

'These are the residues of artificial fertilizers, herbicides and insecticides applied to fields and eaten by cattle, absorbed by grains and left on fruit and vegetables. Nitrates put onto fields drain off into our water supply and antibiotics sometimes fed to poultry and livestock to prevent disease remain in the food chain,' she points out.

The family now buy only organically grown fruit and vegetables, found a butcher who did not feed his animals with chemical hormones and antibiotics and searched out free-range eggs.

Vegetarian, vegan and macrobiotic

For many, the natural progression from many of the diets mentioned so far is a daily menu which not only cuts out meat but also all animal products, and adds more fresh vegetables, fruits and wholefoods.

The vegetarian way of life is becoming more popular anyway, regardless of whether there are illnesses like eczema in the family. Vegetarian restaurants and health food shops are springing up in every high street, and even chain stores have counters where you can buy wholemeal bread, brown sugar, rice and pulses.

The vegan diet takes this a step further, omitting all dairy produce, such as milk, cheese and butter from meals. The macrobiotic diet is even more structured.

All are found to suit and help some people, often controlling or clearing the eczema. Nor does it ever seem too late to try. Terry Tuck who is thirty-seven and has suffered severely from eczema since he was a baby finds his new wholefood diet makes a tremendous difference.

'I was put on a cow's milk-free diet and at the same time had to cut out all animal fats, only eating pork and lamb as meat for meals. I came off white sugar, and now eat more fresh vegetables and fruit. I have soya milk and low fat margarine.

'One thing it improved at once was the very bad night irritation which I had had for many years, and my sleeping was very much better. Now I feel much fitter and eat in a new way. Before, I ate anything that was put in front of me. Now I stick to the wholefood diet, and my skin is clear at present.'

The vegan diet, plus herbal treatment, was the cure for the two young sons of Peter and Helen Tattersall who both suffered from eczema very badly.

The children were put onto a strict vegan diet, starting with a breakfast of soya milk mixed with brown ground rice into a thick sauce with wheat germ, brewer's yeast and kelp powder all containing valuable vitamins and minerals. Lunch was a mixture of lightly cooked vegetables or dishes made with lentils, beans and other pulses.

'For tea they had wholemeal bread sandwiches filled with vegetable spreads, sprouted seeds or vegan cheese made from mixing soyolk flour with melted vegetable margarine. I also made cakes from wholemeal buckwheat and soyolk flour,' explains their mother.

Much of this diet is similar to the macrobiotic, which divides foods for each meal into recommended proportions — at least 50 per cent should be whole cereal grains; 5 per cent special soups and broths with tahini and miso; 25-30 per cent vegetables; and 5-10 per cent beans and sea vegetables.

The diet does not include meat, eggs, animal fat, poultry, dairy products, artificial drinks, tea, coffee or sugar — a useful point to know since many people find that eczema is aggravated by sugar.

Macrobiotic diet also rules out all artificially coloured, preserved, sprayed or chemically treated foods and any hot spices. Food should be eaten calmly and slowly. Macrobiotics, in fact, is a way of life, not just a way of eating.

'We were given a macrobiotic diet for the whole family to follow,' says Justine Marionbanks, mother of a five-year-old with eczema. 'The centre we went to said that it would be too difficult and unfair on David to eat separately.

'So we have been living on brown rice, cereals, peas, beans, grains, green vegetables and seaweed, using miso and soya milk for extra nutrients. It has been a difficult diet, but at least David is getting better.'

This family, like many others, have found they are all feeling healthier for a change in eating habits.

Sample Recipes

MILK-FREE FRUIT ICE CREAM

To 8 oz (225g) of sweetened blackcurrant purée add 2 fl oz (60ml) of
soya milk. Chill in freezer until slushy. Add 1 stiffly beaten egg white,
mix well and return to freezer. (Raspberries and strawberries can also
be used.)

(From Mrs Janet Renwick, printed in *Exchange*.)

SOYA MILK
(makes approx 1½ pints/850 ml)

Imperial (Metric)
5 oz (150g) soya flour
Vanilla pod, honey or concentrated apple juice (optional)

1. Mix flour with 1½ pints (850ml) of water in a saucepan.
2. Bring slowly to the boil, stirring all the time but making sure it
    doesn't froth over. Reduce the heat and simmer for 20 minutes,
    stirring frequently.
3. The milk can be flavoured with honey, apple juice or vanilla pod,
    but add apple juice when milk has cooled as otherwise it may curdle.
    Store in a fridge as mixture ferments when exposed to heat.

(From *The Allergy Diet* by Elizabeth Workman, SRD, Dr John Hunter
and Dr Virginia Alun Jones, Martin Dunitz.)

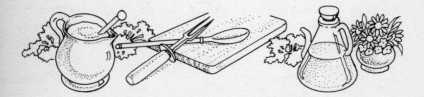

EGG AND MILK-FREE FRUIT CAKE

Imperial (Metric)
1½ oz (45g) almonds, skinned and halved
½ pint (285ml) soya milk (undiluted)
4 fl oz (120ml) water
8 oz (225g) *Tomor* margarine
6 oz (170g) raw cane sugar
1½ lbs (680g) mixed dried fruit
1 orange
Sea salt
Bicarbonate of soda
12 oz (340g) wholewheat cake flour

1. Put milk, water, margarine, sugar and fruit into large saucepan and bring to boil, stirring all the time, then simmer for 15 minutes.
2. Let it cool but not get cold, then add grated rind of orange, pinch of salt, level teaspoon bicarbonate of soda, flour.
3. Mix well, turn into 8 inch (20cm) cake tin (non-stick or well-lined) and decorate top with blanched almonds.
4. Bake in oven for three hours in all, 1 hour at 325°F/170°C (Gas Mark 3) and 2 hours at 275°F/140°C (Gas Mark 1). Cover top with brown paper to prevent nuts burning.

(From a recipe sheet issued by Plantmilk Ltd., the makers of soya milk *Plamil*. They also issue a useful sheet on infant feeding with soya milk, all available from *Plamil* House, Bowles Well Gardens, Dover Road, Folkestone, Kent.)

SPECIAL BAKING POWDER

You can make your own baking powder (raising powder) to make sure that it does not contain wheat-flour or any milk by-product such as lactose.

Imperial (Metric)

¼ oz (7g) potassium bicarbonate
4¾ oz (115g) potato flour (farina)

Mix and store in a screwtop jar. Use as required. Potassium bicarbonate can be bought at chemists.

(From *Wheat-free, Milk-free, Egg-free Cooking* by Rita Greer, Thorsons.)

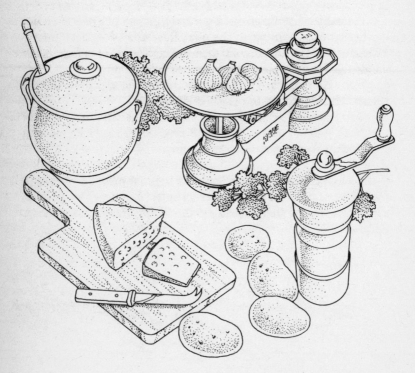

BROWN BREAD FLOUR
Makes 4 loaves

Imperial (Metric)
4 oz (115g) soya flour
1 lb 2 oz (510g) ground brown rice
3 oz (85g) yellow split pea flour
2 tablespoons dried pectin
2 oz (55g) ground almonds
1 heaped tablespoon carob powder

1. Put all ingredients, carefully weighed,* into a large mixing bowl. Mix well, by hand.
2. Put into a polythene bag, seal and use as required. Best stored in the fridge.

*Weights need to be accurate for best results and the imperial measures are the best ones to use.

(From *Wheat-free, Milk-free, Egg-free Cooking.*)

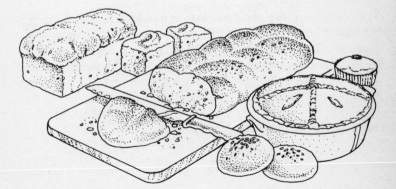

BROWN BREAD

Imperial (Metric)
2 heaped teaspoons dried yeast granules
9 fl oz (250ml) warm water
1 heaped teaspoon raw cane sugar
7¼ oz (210g) brown bread flour
3 pinches sea salt
1 tablespoon sunflower oil

1. Preheat oven at 350°F/180°C (Gas Mark 4).
2. Sprinkle the yeast granules into the warm water. Add the sugar and stir.
3. Leave for a few minutes so that the yeast can soften.
4. Put the flour into a bowl with the sea salt and oil. Mix.
5. Stir the yeast and pour on to the flour.
6. Mix well to a smooth, creamy batter.
7. Grease a loaf tin size 7¼×3½×2¼ in (185×90×50mm) with oil and flour with ground rice or maize flour.
8. Spoon/pour into the prepared tin and put straight into the preheated oven on the top shelf.
9. Bake for about 1 hour, until well risen, brown and crusty.
10. Turn out onto a wire rack to cool as soon as you take it out of the oven. Do not cut until cold as the loaf needs to 'set'.

Note: Use as ordinary bread and store in a polythene bag, sealed. You can make this loaf with fresh yeast — use double the amount given. This loaf is not made or baked in the same way as ordinary bread. As the loaf does not contain gluten the yeast will not behave in the usual way. This is why it does not need to be left to rise and why it is cooked on such a low temperature.

(From *Wheat-free, Milk-free, Egg-free Cooking.*)

ADDITIVE-FREE FISH FINGERS

Imperial (Metric)
12 oz (340g) white fish
Water/Worcestershire sauce
Sea salt and freshly ground black pepper
Fresh wholemeal breadcrumbs from 2 slices bread
12 oz (340g) cooked potato
1 teaspoon margarine

1. Bake the white fish in seasoned water at 375°F/190°C (Gas Mark 5) for 30 minutes.
2. Spread breadcrumbs on a dry baking sheet, season and crisp them in the oven for 10-15 minutes.
3. Flake fish and mash it together with cooked potato, margarine and a little fish stock to moisten. Shape this mixture into fingers, then flatten slightly and square the sides.
4. Roll the fingers on the tray of breadcrumbs. Grill for 15-20 minutes, turning once.

(From *What Can I Give Him Today?* by Diana Wells.)

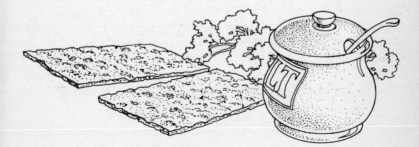

ADDITIVE-FREE SAVOURY PASTIES

Imperial (Metric)

8 oz (225g) shortcrust pastry (using 4 oz (115g) milk-free
  margarine). This is sufficient for 6 pasties, cut with a 4½
  inch (11cm) cutter.

Filling suggestions:

Mince meat with onion, cooked vegetables, tomatoes.
Chicken, mushroom and garlic diced into thick gravy.
Lamb's liver, onion and potato, finely diced.

1. Roll out pastry thinly and cut around a 4½ inch (11cm) disc.
2. Moisten the edges with water, then cover half the pastry circle with
   savoury fillings. Fold in half and seal at edges.
3. Bake at 400°F/200°C (Gas Mark 6) for 25 minutes. These freeze
   well and make quick lunches, teas or nourishing snacks.

(From *What Can I Give Him Today?* by Diana Wells.)

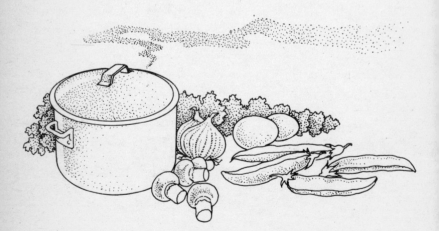

MISO SOUP

Imperial (Metric)
1 onion
1 large carrot
1 small or ½ large head white cabbage
1 tablespoon vegetable oil
3 tablespoons miso paste
2 pints (1.15 litres) water

1. Slice the onions thinly, cut the carrot into matchsticks, and shred the cabbage.
2. Sauté the onions for 2 minutes, then add the carrot and cabbage and sauté them for 5-10 minutes longer, stirring constantly.
3. Add the water, bring to the boil and simmer for 20 minutes.
4. Remove some of the liquid and mix it in a cup with the miso paste until the paste is dissolved. Add this to the soup, mix thoroughly and serve.

(From *Vegan Cooking* by Leah Leneman, Thorsons.)

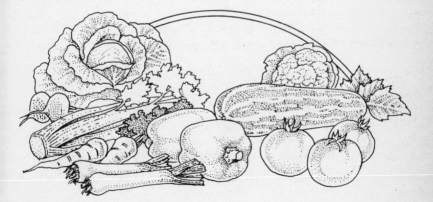

CAULIFLOWER AND OAT BAKE

Imperial (Metric)
1 medium onion, grated
1 teaspoon yeast extract
4 oz (115g) rolled oats
2 oz (55g) button mushrooms, chopped
1 small cauliflower, broken into small florets and lightly
  cooked
2 eggs, separated.
Seasoning
1 oz (28g) medium fat cheese, grated (optional)

1. Cook the onion in the yeast extract until tender.
2. Mix with the oats, mushrooms, cauliflower florets, beaten egg yolks and seasoning.
3. Stiffly beat the egg whites and fold into the vegetables.
4. Pile into a baking dish, top with cheese and bake at 375°F/190°C (Gas Mark 5) for 35-40 minutes.

(From *The Vegetarian on a Diet* by Jill Metcalfe and Margaret Cousins, Thorsons.)

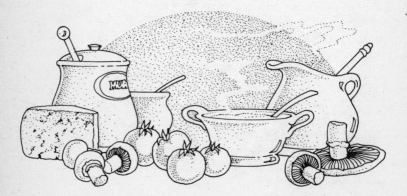

RICE AND BEAN BURGERS

Imperial (Metric)
2 tablespoons vegetable oil
1 leek
Approximately 4 oz (115g) cooked kidney beans (or others)
8 oz (225g) cooked brown rice
Mixed herbs
Soya sauce
Rolled oats
Vegetable oil for frying

1. Heat 2 tablespoons of oil and add the finely chopped leek. Cook until transparent.
2. Remove from the heat and mash the beans into the leeks. Then combine this mixture with the rice, herbs and soya sauce. If the mixture is too dry, add some water or stock.
3. Form into burgers and roll in the oats. Fry on both sides.

(From *Simple and Speedy Wholefood Cooking* by Janet Hunt, Thorsons.)

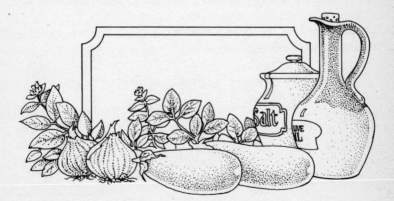

HOME-BAKED BEANS

The taste of home-baked beans is enough to put you off the tinned variety for life. This recipe can be served either as a main course, perhaps topped with cheese or served with jacket potatoes, or as an accompaniment.

Imperial (Metric)

8 oz (225g) haricot beans, soaked overnight
1 large onion, sliced
1 tablespoon oil
1 teaspoon mustard powder
2 teaspoons molasses
2 tablespoons tomato purée
2 teaspoons Muscovado sugar
¾ pint (375ml) stock
2 tablespoons cider vinegar

1. Drain the beans. Cook in boiling water for about an hour (or 15 minutes in a pressure cooker) until almost tender.
2. Fry the onion in the oil for 5 minutes, add the rest of the ingredients and the drained beans, and bring to the boil.
3. Cover and cook at 275°F/140°C (Gas Mark 1) for 4 hours, stirring occasionally. This recipe freezes well.

(From *The Healthy Baby Cookbook* by Carol Hunter, Thorsons.)

For further recipes, see the suggested books mentioned here, or those listed on pages 151-2.

The Whole View

There are two main reasons why so many eczema sufferers have been turning to so-called 'fringe' medicine in recent years. The first is that they feel a desperate need to find an alternative to the steroid treatments so often prescribed by the orthodox medical profession. The second is that they have seen evidence these alternative therapies actually work. In fact the words 'fringe' and 'alternative' aren't any longer particularly apt, since many of the therapies are no longer seen as outside the realms of orthodox medicine but very much a part of it.

More widely used nowadays is the phrase 'complementary' medicine, which accurately reflects the growing movement to encourage all those in the health field to work together and learn from each other.

'Natural' and 'holistic' are also both excellent descriptions of the various methods used and the general approach. The accent in treatment is always on the natural ways to help the body heal itself and maintain health — and the person is seen as a whole, not simply as a collection of symptoms.

Personality, temperament, eating habits, lifestyle, general health and illness, all should be taken into account before a diagnosis is made and treatment recommended.

Nor are the various therapies seen as totally separate from each other. Many are interdependent, or overlap, so that homoeopathic remedies may be combined with acupuncture, and herbal cures used alongside osteopathy and massage. Diet is an underlying factor of them all, as part of the general philosophy that symptoms must be treated from the inside of the person, rather than suppressed from the outside.

The therapies are also seen as preventive. Instead of waiting to be ill and then doing something about it, the idea is that you live your life in such a way that illness is kept at bay, with body and mind functioning harmoniously together.

These are the ideals, anyway, and it isn't surprising that after the boom years of drug use and abuse, with a pill or new miracle cream the apparent answer to every ache and pain, that there is renewed interest in more natural ways to health. Having been considered somewhat cranky and peculiar, holistic medicine is growing in popularity again.

Ancient therapies

What *is* surprising is that natural medicine should be seen in certain quarters as new-fangled and part of a rather trendy fashion, since most of the therapies are extremely ancient in origin.

Some formed the foundation of today's orthodox medicine, their methods based on theories and substances which should be approved of by modern medical science.

For instance, many of today's drugs are still derived from plants, such as *digitalis* from foxgloves, which is used to treat heart disorder. *Urtia dioica*, better known to us as stinging nettle, was used by the Romans against chills and skin disorders — a very logical remedy when analysis shows it to contain a substance similar to histamine.

The various spas, rich in mineral waters, have long been known to help all sorts of disorders, including skin conditions, and the Victorians trooped to these centres in their hundreds. Acupuncture and many other therapies are a respected part of traditional Eastern medicine.

Of course, some of the therapies are easier to accept than others, particularly in these days when a practical explanation and solid proof is wanted before anything can be believed.

The cleansing diet of naturopathy which seeks to rid the body of toxic substances to promote health and heal illness makes sense if you think about it. So do the therapeutic effects of herbs, particularly when you bear in mind that for centuries they were the only source of treatment.

Homoeopathy also adds up, the theory behind it being to treat 'like with like', in a sense akin to immunization which protects the body from various illnesses by actually causing the illness on a minor scale so that the body builds up immunity.

Less easy to understand and explain are the therapies such as acupuncture, reflexology and radionics, which deal with the energy currents in the body and are as much spiritual and mental as physical.

But, since the mysteries of the human make-up in general, and of conditions like eczema in particular, are so mysterious anyway, still shrouded in all sorts of enigmas, such therapies should not be dismissed out of hand, particularly when the proof of the pudding can be in the eating.

For some people acupuncture, faith healing, dowsing and all the other more inexplicable therapies have worked, whether or not anyone understands why or can give a logical explanation in everyday language.

Justified doubts

Sometimes doubts are justified and people do feel wary of trying certain branches of natural medicine, or are very disappointed when they have done so. Even then it may be fairer to blame the practitioner rather than the method, since it is still too easy for unqualified people to set themselves up as 'trained' therapists.

All sorts of individuals, organizations and manufacturers can make wild claims that they can cure eczema and then lead patients and their families on a wild goose chase that may end in disillusionment and disappointment.

Writes one man who has had eczema all his life, and has been caught out in the past: 'It seems that there are those who are prepared to trade on those of us who suffer from eczema even to the extent of creating dependence on it in their professed claims of service and products — i.e., a recent ad in our local paper which recommended sunbeds as having "therapeutic healing benefits" for sufferers from eczema.

'My concern is that if at all possible we should be able to safeguard and protect ourselves from spurious beliefs, pseudo cures, fake claims and so on. We can ill-afford them, even those that appear well-intentioned.'

A very worried mother of a two-year-old girl wrote to me following her experience with a particular clinic which she found from an advert in a health magazine. Her daughter was put on a stone-age diet with no dairy products, additives, beef, pork, wheat, cereals, colouring and certain fruits.

'She also had various homoeopathic medicines and was on bottled water,' says her mother. 'But apart from a less clingy and fractious tendency in her nature, the eczema was the same. Then, after thirteen weeks a hair analysis was taken and this revealed a calcium deficiency.

'The therapist herself had given me the report to take home and read to save the money of her reading it in consultation time! So I stopped the diet without first consulting her as I was frightened of a two-year-old being short of calcium. When I rang and told the clinic they said she should have got enough from vegetables, but in fact she wouldn't eat vegetables, and in the end was only eating meat.'

Quite apart from these dietery deficiencies and the lack of proper guidance and advice, this mother was worried about the cost of private fees and special foods, and also the general disruption of family life.

'Did the financial and emotional strain on the family cause as much trauma and tension as the eczema did and does?' she asks. 'Our daughter has not got very severe eczema but we tried every avenue for a cure we could find because you always feel "is this the treatment that's going to work?"'

Rather as mentioned in the chapters on diet, it is possible to get caught on a treadmill, frantically experimenting with one therapy after another, perhaps never quite carrying any of them through thoroughly enough or finding the best and most reputable practitioners, and suffering even more as a consequence.

The difficulty is that often experimentation is necessary because of the variable nature of eczema. Some people are lucky and hit upon the right therapy straight away. Other people must shop around and try various methods before they find any relief.

Also as mentioned in the introduction to this book, because eczema fluctuates anyway, and quite often an adult or child has a remission which lasts for long periods or even a lifetime, it can be difficult to assess results.

So, as important as anything else is the attitude of mind when deciding to attempt a particular therapy. Though it is essential to be as thorough and dedicated as possible, it is also necessary to keep a fairly philosophical frame of mind and not become too obsessed or cast down if, in the end, there is little improvement.

Finding a practitioner

It is also important to find properly trained practitioners and therapists. In spite of the growing popularity of natural methods, it isn't always easy to discover what is available and where. Therapies are mostly available privately, and can be expensive, with practitioners difficult to locate.

This is where many of the organizations set up to train and co-ordinate the methods of the various therapies can be very helpful. There are now associations and societies for almost all of them, including naturopathy, osteopathy, herbalism, homoeopathy, reflexology, acupuncture and radionics. Names and addresses are given in the final section of this book.

Other organizations are acting as co-ordinators of the various therapies, bringing together the strands that make up the complete picture of holistic medicine. An example of this is the Natural Health Network which links natural health centres and interested individuals all over the country.

Many of the centres have a group of practitioners of different therapies working under the same roof, and they meet together for workshops and training sessions, and have a newsletter with names and addresses of the various members.

Other organizations are being set up as a type of watchdog body enquiring into the reliability and safety of certain therapies. For instance, the British Medical Association on Alternative Therapies is an an enquiry into training and practice, but has been criticized for being too medically centred with few actual practitioners taking part.

'Unfortunately the BMA are looking for scientific explanations of all therapies — what they cannot prove they will not believe,' says an issue of the Natural Health Network newsletter. 'Sadly the application of scientific methods to prove that natural therapies work will produce little more than nonsense. Healing, and to some measure the other complementary methods, are outside the scope of current textbooks.'

But the Network sees it as healthy that orthodox medics should be taking such an interest in a subject that so many once considered taboo. Further proof of this was the setting up of the British Holistic Medical Association, which seeks to educate and train doctors and medical students in accepting and understanding natural therapies.

More recently the Council for Alternative and Complementary Medicine has been formed, this time by the various alternative organizations themselves, including the British Acupuncture Association, the National Institute of Medical Herbalists and the British Naturopathic and Osteopathic Association.

The Council states its aim 'is to promote and maintain the highest standards of training, qualification and treatment in complementary and alternative medicine . . . The Council is deeply concerned with the safety of the public and committed to the principle that all those who practise non-orthodox medicine are ethically controlled and bound by codes of practice.'

Yet another umbrella group is the Institute for Complementary Medicine, which again seeks to standardize the training of all practitioners in all therapies so that qualifications are uniform, rather than varying as they do now from one individual to another.

The Institute also has what it calls Public Information Points round the country which are manned by volunteers who can give information on therapies, arrange public classes and lectures and suggest suitable local clinics and practitioners.

Diagnosis by radionics
Most of the natural therapies have their own particular forms of diagnosis, much of this depending on in-depth discussion with the patient which takes account not just of the symptoms of illness but also of all sorts of details about personality, temperament, medical history and lifestyle.

The state of eyes and nails would be examined, a urine sample, blood-pressure and pulse rate taken and, in certain cases, X-rays made, much as in an orthodox medical examination.

But certain types of diagnosis, for instance analysis using blood sample, saliva or a lock of hair, are not only part of a particular therapy with its own healing methods, but can be used in conjunction with other therapies, too.

An example of this is radionics. Though a form of diagnosis and therapy which is often dismissed as decidedly odd and suspect by some, there is an association of radionic practitioners, and a great many followers who believe in its authenticity and benefits.

Radionics is based on the theory that energy patterns are emitted by all forms of matter, including the human body, and with the use of various instruments — for instance the 'black box' — it is possible for the practitioner to identify and measure any distortions or disharmonies in these patterns.

'All disharmonies have a cause and all causes are recognizable by their own particular energy patterns,' explains the Radionics Association. 'Frequently there is one basic cause or factor which is fundamental to ill health. When this is identified and corrected, the curative work is then completed by the patient's own natural healing forces.

'To a radionic practitioner, a patient's named disease or symptoms are like the visible tip of an iceberg, the remaining unseen part of the iceberg representing deeper levels of the patient's being — the energy levels — of which he is totally unaware.'

As the association points out, it is not even necessary for the patient to be present. Blood, hair or saliva sample will be used for diagnosis, and treatment can be effective whether patient and practitioner are in the same room or at opposite ends of the earth!

But they also stress that not all patients respond to radionics and sometimes an additional or alternative treatment will be recommended, such as change in diet, osteopathic or chiropractic manipulation, homoeopathic or herbal remedies or a referral back to the GP. Although it is not widely known, some doctors and specialists use radionic practitioners for diagnosis, including confirmation of allergies.

One woman who was treated by radionics expresses her original scepticism when a friend recommended this therapy to treat a red, patchy rash from which she was suffering. Like many others, she thought it all sounded highly unbelievable.

'I very much dislike and mistrust anything in the nature of quack cures,' she writes. 'But after a few weeks my mother persuaded me that it could do no harm so I chewed a piece of cotton wool, sent it to the doctor concerned, and forgot all about it.

'I received some pills (I think homoeopathic) and a diet sheet. I took some pills and had my first tolerable night in weeks. No fresh patches developed and my skin cleared up quickly.'

In spite of similar misgivings about the strange-sounding method, the mother of a little boy with eczema took him to a radionic practitioner to diagnose food allergies.

'Since then I have carefully followed the diet she gave me even though it was quite a difficult and restricted one,' says this mother. 'Slowly Julian has improved and become a changed baby. He can play on his own or happily watch me for quite long periods without scratching, even though his skin is still a bit blotchy in places.'

Diagnosis by dowsing

Dowsing is an equally mysterious form of diagnosis. Although it has its own practitioners and association, The British Society of Dowsers, this therapy works on the same theory of energy patterns as radionics and is often practised by the same people.

But instead of a box or other panel of instruments, the dowser will use a pendulum or stick and interpret diagnosis by the movements of this in response to changes in the brain rythms and muscular responses of the body. Water divining and metal detection is another branch of dowsing, and works on a similar principle.

According to the British Society of Dowsers and others I have spoken to, anyone can have the ability to dowse successfully. But the essential requirement is that both dowser and patient must have belief and faith in what is happening.

To try for yourself, a pendulum can be made by hanging a large bead from a thin cord about 1 foot (30cm) long. Learn to swing the pendulum over the body by starting it deliberately. Either it will go straight left-to-right; to and fro away from the body; or in clockwise or anti-clockwise circles.

To interpret the pendulum's answers to specific questions one practitioner suggests holding it over a coin and asking 'Is this a coin?' The answer must be 'yes', so you note the swing and enter it as the answer for 'yes'. Ask whether the coin is a piece of cheese and you should get the pendulum swing meaning 'no', and so on.

After this you move on to specific questions such as: 'Is there an allergy to milk?' or 'Is there allergy to eggs?' and note the answer in the swing. I must say I remain sceptical, but one herbalist in Cambridge has assured me that she has seen some surprising results. Allergies diagnosed by the pendulum swing have been proved right since subsequent dieting and changes in lifestyle have cleared the eczema.

Successful treatment

But perhaps I should leave the last word in this chapter with a patient, and one who has found radionics and many other forms of natural therapy a great help in keeping her eczema at bay.

Writes Vivien Anderson: 'I had small patches of eczema as a baby and in my teens the patches flared up from time to time. I was given *Betnovate* cream which I used on and off for 10 years or so. After marriage my eczema became even more noticeable, my hands were raw, cracked and bleeding.

'I went to see my local GP, whom I had rarely consulted. He didn't think I needed a skin specialist as I requested, did no tests, but offered more cream and a prescription for pills which I later found were *Valium*. I left the surgery refusing the cream and the pills.'

It was after this that Vivien decided to try alternatives, and visited clinics she saw advertised in a health magazine. The first was not satisfactory, but the second, she says, was like a haven.

'The approach was confident but calm, the atmosphere relaxed yet professional. I was told I would need a fair amount of treatment from the various practitioners at the clinic and would have to take responsiblity for my own health by avoiding unnecessary drugs and following a diet.'

Vivien filled in a detailed form, and a week later had a session of radionic analysis. Homoeopathic and herbal remedies, vitamin and mineral supplements and a soothing cream and lotion (*calendula*) were prescribed, and she was shown how to cleanse her skin with a friction rub which stimulated circulation.

'In addition I had some acupuncuture (very relaxing) and my pulses were taken in Chinese fashion, as an aid to diagnosis. I was warned I could expect to become worse before I became better, as my body threw off the toxic matter in my system. I began my cleansing diet, gradually introducing new foods and eliminating others.'

The treatment followed the pattern of acupuncture, spinal adjustment and attention to the pelvis (osteopathy) and once a month there was radionic analysis to note changes in the system and adjust remedies.

'As I improved my treatment sessions became less frequent,' says Vivien. 'My skin became clear gradually — one year later it was completely clear. I now have radionic analysis once a year — I call it my MOT and discuss any problems I have.

'My husband and family are very sceptical about it all but my reply is: "The proof of the pudding . . ." If it works, keep doing it. I am just grateful for the health I enjoy today.'

The Nature Cure

Naturopathy is a distinct holistic therapy in its own right. Because its underlying philosphy embodies much of what the whole field of natural medicine is about, the name is often used as an umbrella to cover other therapies as well.

Even though the term naturopathy was first heard at the turn of this century, many of the healing methods date back to 400 B.C. when Hippocrates treated disease in accordance with natural laws. As the British Naturopathic and Oesteopathic Association explains, there are three main principles on which these are based.

The first is that the body possesses the power to heal itself through its inborn intelligence and vitality. The second is that the symptoms of disease are the manifestation of this vital force applying itself to the removal of toxins, stress and imbalance in the body.

The third principle is that the causes and effects of disease are not simply located in an isolated organ or system, but arise out of a person's lifestyle.

'Each individual responds in unique ways to his or her environment,' says the Association. 'Reactions to the same stress may be very different depending on the level of mental and bodily health, inherited tendencies and previous medical history. In treating the whole person, the naturopath searches for causes of illness on many and interacting levels.'

As he points out, these could be biochemical — i.e., an imbalance in the chemistry of the body fluids owing to dietary deficiencies or excess, or a retention of waste products in the body.

Causes can also be mechanical and connected with muscular injury, or postular stress which leads in turn to interference with the correct functioning of the nervous system. This is why osteopathy often plays a useful part in naturopathic treatments.

Finally the Association mentions psychological stress, with the practitioner looking at the person's anxieties and pressures in personal, domestic and professional life, and with an awareness of how much stress can manifest itself physically.

The first visit to a naturopath will usually last forty-five minutes or so, and involves taking a detailed medical case history and thorough physical examination, possibly with X-rays or blood tests.

Treatment, once diagnosis has been made, will include other therapies such as osteopathy and hydrotherapy, but will also recommend a balanced lifestyle with plenty of physical exercise, relaxation and the cultivation of a positive approach to life and health.

Naturopathy and eczema

These, then, are the general principles of naturopathy. To find out how these apply to eczema I talked to Ray Hill who practises naturopathy — or nature cure as he prefers to call it — in Nottingham.

He, like many other naturopaths, has a simplistic view of the treatment of eczema, built up over many years of personal experience. He maintains that the skin, an eliminative organ, is being overworked as a result of other organs of elimination not functioning adequately.

Using iridology, a form of diagnosis which studies the iris of the eyes, Ray Hill says that the skin area on the edge of the iris always shows signs of congestion — and in most instances so does the bowel area.

'My argument is that the toxic condition of the bowel is the principal reason for many of the skin conditions suffered by man,' he explains. 'But obviously the lungs, kidneys and lymph systems must be considered, too. And only when all eliminative organs are working in balance, taking their fair share of the load, can these skin complaints heal.

'So my first consideration is the use of herbs to begin the cleansing process. I use a formula passed down to me from one of the early pioneers of nature cure which is called *Vitalax*. These herbs have been specially combined to work in cleansing the liver, kidneys, bowels, lungs and skin.

'Ninety per cent of all disease starts with the bowel. And unless a person has two or three bowel movements daily, they must be considered constipated. Animals defecate after every meal and humans should too! The amount of waste stored in the bowel of constipated people has to be seen to be believed.

'All the time it is there, every hour of the day, the fluid and toxic waste matter is being absorbed back into the system to be deposited in another part of the body according to one's inherent weaknesses. The other eliminative organs have to cope with the extra load in a desperate effort to keep the body's functions working.'

It is for this reason that Ray Hill says eczema is the result of an internal toxic condition and any treatment must start with internal cleansing. To use creams and ointments alone, he maintains, is simply a waste of time and money, particularly as those normally prescribed by orthodox practitioners actually inhibit real healing. Cosmetically they may be effective, but the cause has not been dealt with, and until it is a naturally clear skin isn't possible.

The cleansing diet

Diet plays an enormous part in Ray Hill's treatment, and foods have been categorized by him under three headings — cleansing, nourishing and congesting.

According to the toxic condition of the patient, so the diet is planned. At the beginning he cuts out the congesting foods (heavy proteins, carbohydrates and junk foods), reduces the nourishing foods (leafy and root vegetables) and increases the cleansing foods (fruits).

'The introduction of congesting foods comes later,' he says, 'but these are always limited. I would not expect people to go back to their original eating habits, because it was that and the poor elimination which was the main cause of the eczema in the first place.'

On the question of emotional and mental experiences causing skin conditions, Ray Hill thinks there are two main factors. First, in his opinion, the body is too impoverished with a junk diet to have the vitality to cope with some nervous or emotional upheavals.

He also thinks that some people are conditioned to think wrongly and therefore meet a particularly harrowing experience with the wrong attitude. 'The response then causes a physical flare-up. The fact that emotional feeling can affect the skin is very easily seen by blushing. It is possible, by a change of thinking, to stop oneself blushing.'

He also has very strong feelings about infantile eczema, believing that the cause lies in the parent's toxic condition which has been passed on to the baby. He feels, too, that if one continues to feed an eczematic child with milk and milk products, it is almost inevitable that asthma or bronchial problems will occur later in life.

'Eradicating milk from the diet in this situation certainly reduces the possibility of asthma later and can help the skin condition immediately,' he points out. 'This is because cow's milk is a congesting food and not good for children.

'It is designed for bovine creatures and simply causes the eliminative organs to overwork, especially the lymphatic system. This is why children get swollen tonsils and adenoids. Cut out the milk, introduce fruit juices, and the enlarged glands subside, because the pressure on them has been reduced.

'Feeding cereals to babies before the system has developed sufficiently to deal with them properly is another cause of skin problems and other conditions, particularly later in life. This is one of the reasons, I think, why so many people nowadays appear to have allergies.'

Ray Hill's views are radical, but they appear to have stood the test of time and he, along with other nature cure practitioners, has had success in clearing eczema once people have been persuaded to choose a different diet.

'It's up to the individuals,' says Ray Hill. 'We can show the way, but they have to do it themselves. There are no wonder pills or lotions which will cure. It is only by careful assessment of each individual, and then the balancing of assimalation and elimination that you get long-lasting results.

'But the work, effort and attitude of the patient is the real difference between success and failure. In the end it is he or she who has to be willing to make the changes.'

Patients' experience
Certainly many children and adults with eczema have experienced good results from naturopathy, often combining it with other therapies. One

of the most unforgettable cases I have known is that of the Tattersall family, whose vegan diet was included in Chapter 6.

When I first met Peter and Helen Tattersall, their little boy Kevin was two years old and covered in eczema from head to foot. His parents had forgotten what it was like to have an unbroken night of sleep, often getting up five or six times to attend to Kevin.

When their second son was born and showed signs of eczema, they didn't feel they could cope any more. They had already experimented with diet unsuccessfully, including goat's milk, and had been to many different specialists. But the breakthrough came when they visited a naturopath and herbalist in Manchester, recommended to them by someone whose child had made a remarkable recovery after treatment.

'He took a blood analysis and prescribed herbal drops and creams,' remembers Helen. 'He also advised us to keep Kevin on a strict vegan diet, with no animal fats or produce at all. So we replaced cow's milk with soya bean substitute and read more books on the subject.'

When Peter and Helen took Kevin to the naturopath he told them they were not to expect instant results but that eventually he would have skin like velvet. After a year that's exactly what he had, and his baby brother did too — something which I saw with my own eyes.

This family felt they were helped by the fact their children were so young, but adults with a life-time of eczema have also found naturopathy has eased and even cleared their symptoms.

'For the past two years I have been receiving treatment for my eczema from a naturopathic practitioner with acupuncture, homoeopathy, osteopathy and special diet included,' writes a young mother in *Exchange*. 'While not completely cured, the eczema is under control and I only have a couple of small patches which appear in autumn — my low season.

'I saw an advert in a health magazine and decided to have a go. First I had acupuncture and osteopathic treatment, and began a special diet, 60-70 per cent of which had to be fruit and vegetables, raw or lightly steamed, 10 per cent carbohydrates and fats. I was prescribed homoeopathic tablets and an iron tonic. Since then I have returned for treatments and check-ups as necessary.

'I particularly appreciated the practitioner's attitude — for the first time my rash was being taken seriously. As that improved, so did my state of mind and I became stronger. When the eczema had been clear for while, I decided to become pregnant and stayed with the practitioner for all treatment.

'I felt very fit throughout my pregnancy, worked almost to the end and had to move house a few days before the baby arrived. I am convinced that I had I not been receiving this treatment, I would not have been able to cope as I did.'

Uses of osteopathy

This patient, like many others receiving naturopathic treatment, was given osteopathy. Because many people simply think of osteopaths as putting backs and bones generally 'back into place' the relevance of this therapy to eczema is not always obvious.

But in fact osteopathy is based on the concept of wholeness of the body and mind. If there is an imbalance or disturbance in the mechanical structure, the body functions will be under strain. If the body structure is in correct alignment, then the nerve and blood systems of the body are free to protect, build, repair and restore.

In a very useful booklet which they produce, The General Council and Register of Osteopaths explains that the forms of treatment used after diagnosis has been made are mostly manipulative in character.

'The types and severity of mechanical derangements are numerous in example and vary greatly, as do the effects which they have on the human body,' explains the Council. 'Those that occur in the vicinity of the spine are thought by osteopaths to have a special significance because of the close relationship of the spine to the distributive channels of the nervous system.

'Through this association of the spine and the nervous system there has emerged in the teaching of osteopathy a belief that mechanical derangements caused through injury and stress to the fabric of the spine matter to one's health both in a general and specific way, due to the influence they can have on parts of the nervous system. As time goes by there is more and more evidence to show that this approach has a sound basis.'

Osteopath and naturopath Jeanette Thomson has used these therapies, plus homoeopathic and mineral treatments, to help many patients, including her own husband who suffered badly from eczema when she first met him.

'Most eczema sufferers believe that skin problems are just related to the skin itself, and don't realize that the whole of the body is responsible for the skin's well-being,' she says. 'The skin shouldn't be looked at in isolation, as its healthy and efficient working depends upon the way the body as a whole is functioning.

'To be healthy the skin needs a good blood supply, and skin sufferers often find that osteopathic treatment for some unrelated back or structural condition clears up a long-standing skin ailment. For instance, if the body is not used adequately because of insufficient exercise, the tissues will become sluggish and subsequently clogged with toxins.

'Equally, tension caused by the stress of modern living can make muscles become too tense, and any change in the muscle tone can lead to problems in the body's main support system, the spine, causing a bone to become slightly misplaced resulting in pressure on nerves and interference with the blood supply.

'Once this happens the body is unable to function properly, resulting in many ailments such as pain, swelling, and breathing and skin problems. The oesteopath's aim, therefore, is to correct any muscle or bone problems so that the body can restore itself to good health.'

Chiropractic

Osteopathy is better known than chiropractic in this country, even by the layman who has little knowledge of most holistic therapies. Yet chiropractic is based on similar theories to osteopathy, working on the belief that mechanical disorders of the joints can affect the nervous system and therefore the whole body and its health.

However, the British Chiropractic Association whilst agreeing that there are similarities between the two therapies, point out some important differences.

'Chiropractors make use of direct adjustment of a specific vertebra in a given direction, whereas osteopaths often use more massage or soft tissue techniques during the treatment of patients,' the Association explains.

'Also chiropractors use X-rays more frequently than osteopaths and also make fuller use of other diagnostic tests. The early osteopaths believed that the effect of their treatment was on the blood circulation whereas chiropractors emphasized, and still do, the role of the nervous system.'

Many disorders which would appear at first glance to have nothing to do with bones or structure have been helped by chiropractic, including asthma, migraine, digestive disorders and constipation. Patient experience has also shown it has its uses for eczema, often alongside other therapies.

Writes the mother of five-year-old Clare who had a great deal of success with mineral therapy when she took her daughter to a homoeopath: 'I also took Clare to a chiropractor who found that certain bones in her spine were very much out of alignment, especially around the bottom of the neck where asthma and eczema can be centred. She has had four sessions with him and her spine has responded well and is settling into the correct position.

'This treatment is done every three weeks for an hour at a time at a cost of £5 per session and is completely painless. In fact she thoroughly enjoys it. Clare's skin is now clearing following this and the homoeopathic mineral treatment. She is now very, very happy and bright, and is doing well at school.'

Nature cure clinics

With the growing general interest in natural therapies, health hydros and nature cure clinics are becoming increasingly popular again. Seen for a time as either cranky or as smart places for the rich, many more people are realizing the benefit of an intensive health cure for a body which has been ill-treated by the over-indulgence and stress of modern life.

At such clinics it is possible for the first time to experience the effects of naturopathic treatments on the body but practitioners believe that, for the full benefits to be felt, it is necessary to adopt a new lifestyle long term.

A weekend of fasting, fruit juice and exercise may make you feel a lot better and give clues to possible food intolerance and other problems but, when coping with a condition like eczema, you have got to take what you learn back into everyday life for it to really work.

One nature clinic in Edinburgh is modelled very much on the old-style where it is recognized that an improvement in health can only come about from a change in habits. This clinic sees its visitors falling into two main categories:

'There are those who are jaded and out of condition, and recognize their need to regain fitness through self-discipline, and those with recurrent or long-standing illnesses for whom the main need is intensive personal guidance towards a completely reformed way of life.

'Human illnesses result from many factors, so our attention must be correspondingly wide in scope. Psychological understanding may be as vital as physical readjustment, and the aim is to provide a balance between three primary aspects of human existence — physical, mental and ethical.

'The practice involves balanced and restorative diets and spinal and other manipulative adjustments, with general and remedial exercises to suit the patients. Much importance is attached to emotional readjustment. These, together with sunlight and various forms of water treatment — the foundation stones of nature cure — are the main methods.'

Water treatment, or hydrotherapy, is frequently used at clinics and can be particularly beneficial for skin disorders such as eczema. Hydrotherapy can cleanse the pores, improve the circulation and ease the underlying muscle tone.

Treatments available at many clinics and hydros include Sitz baths, where the patient bathes alternately in hot and cold hip-baths; Scottish Douche in which alternating jets of hot and cold water stimulate the spinal column; and salt water and mineral baths. Almost all centres have swimming pools, many with jacuzzis which play jets of water onto the body underwater, providing exercise, relaxation and toning muscles.

Wax and mud baths, Faradic electrical muscle stimulation, saunas and steam cabinets, body massage by hand or vibrator, or with the use of aromatic oils (aromatherapy), plus acupuncture, osteopathy, meditation and yoga are all treatments found at clinics which could help the eczema sufferer.

Diet will, as always, be an underlying link for every therapy, and special diets are catered for. Though not as common as it used to be, fasting is also a part of naturopathy and at a clinic this can be carried out under controlled conditions with the help of people who know— or should know — what they are doing.

But one word of warning — modern health clinics take many forms and it is necessary to find out a great deal about aims, methods and cost before making a choice. Some centres are big business, cashing in on the general trend towards healthier living and the desperate need for help felt by some with chronic conditions.

Parading under all sorts of names, including beauty farms and purification centres, some charge enormous sums of money for services which could be found at a much higher standard and for far less money elsewhere.

So make careful enquiries, perhaps with one of the natural health organizations listed at the end of this book, and send for details of facilities and prices before signing on the dotted line.

Herbs for Health

Herbalism is one of the most ancient of therapies — in fact as old as medicine itself. Man has been using herbs, roots and flowers for the relief of disease for at least 5,000 years.

All ancient civilizations have records of the use of herbs in the treatment of common illnesses. In 450 B.C. Hippocrates was recommending senna as a purgative, and today so many centuries later this herbal remedy is still prescribed.

A large number of plants qualify as medicinal. About 250 are legally entitled to be administered, but far more can be helpful. Although not officially recognized, other remedies passed down through the generations are in use today and people still gather herbs from garden and hedgerows, making up their own preparations.

Says one adult sufferer from eczema: 'A growing interest in all things natural led me to investigate herbal remedies and I discovered that there was a wealth of herbs and plants which are recommended as cures of eczema.

'I was determined to make my own ointments though I knew very little of plants at that time — so little, in fact, that when one book of herbal remedies recommended Plantain my immediate reaction was to wonder where I could buy it, little realizing that I spent half my life tramping on the stuff.'

Another adult with eczema found great relief from a comfrey and marigold healing cream made up at home by a herbalist who used herbs fresh from the garden, plus sunflower and coconut oil. 'The overall effect was to greatly reduce irritation,' she says, 'and also the unsightly redness of the affected areas. The relief I can only describe as wonderful.'

In her book *The Home Herbal* Barbara Griggs describes many home-brewed remedies for eczema. She recommends using red clover, bright orange marigold and the violet flowers and leaves of the heartsease to make infusions, adding a teaspoon of the dried herbs to a cupful of boiling water for ten minutes, stirring and then straining. This should be drunk three times a day.

Stinging nettles are also very effective, she says. The young tops should be picked off the plant from a spot where they are not contaminated by drifting pesticides or pollution from passing cars and made into tea by infusing a dessertspoonful to a cup of boiling water for ten minutes.

Many herbs can also be bought over the counter from herbal shops, health stores and some chemists, either dried or made up into infusions, ointments and tablets. Most manufacturers of toiletries now include herbal preparations in their range.

Professional help

Self-treatment has its drawbacks, though. Home-made creams and ointments are easily contaminated, and herbal remedies need to be made up in exactly the right way for full benefits to be gained. It is not one ingredient in the herb but the whole plant acting in harmony, each part supporting and balancing the other, that has the good effect.

Also, it is not so much for the illness but the causes and symptoms that one herb is recommended more than another. Because of this, and the importance of correct diagnosis, most herbal enthusiasts prefer to consult a professional medical herbalist who has studied the subject in depth and can safely recommend the right herb for the right disorder.

Explains a spokesman for the National Institute of Medical Herbalists: 'Herbs have different properties from drugs, and are therefore applied in their own way. Instead of attacking the symptoms of the disease as drugs do (such as cough, pain or stiffened joints) herbs are suited to supporting the body's own attempts to solve the problem.

'This means actually finding out why the symptoms are there. The herbalist sees the body as capable of looking after itself under normal circumstances, and diseases as a sign that the body has failed to cope in some way, and is desperately, sometimes painfully, trying to compensate. Herbs are ideal for helping the body to get over its adversity in specific ways.

'Because the herbalist treats the whole person, rather than the symptoms, the name of the disease being suffered is of less importance than it is in conventional medicine. Sometimes the apparently trivial complaint is harder to treat than something that looks formidable at first glance — it all depends on the resources available for recovery in each individual, and how easily they may be tapped by treatment.'

So if three people with arthritis see a medical herbalist, they will each go out with a different prescription because they are all individuals who have developed arthritis for different reasons.

To be able to apply herbs correctly means that the herbalist must be well-trained in the medical skills of diagnosis and prescriptions, and the treatment of chronic and complex conditions is best done by someone with training and experience.

In fact, there are fairly strict rules laid down on the diagnosis of illness and use of herbal remedies, so that certain serious conditions are not thought suitable for this type of therapy.

But some herbalists are also trained in other branches of holistic medicine so that along with herbs they may also prescribe naturopathy, acupuncture or osteopathy. Most will also pay a lot of attention to diet, and also any emotional conflicts in a patient's life, perhaps suggesting solutions.

Herbs for eczema

Thomas Bartram is also a member of the National Institute of Medical Herbalists and during his years of practice has had many successes treating the eczema of young babies, children and adults.

'Most children have a touch of eczema sometime during their lives,' he says. 'The older generation of herbalists believe this is due to the presence of cellulites, or accumulated toxins, transmitted at birth and now working their way out of the body. They would prescribe powerful lymphatic and blood tonics.

'In treating eczema my first thought as a herbalist would be skin care from the inside using specific herbal medicines or herbal teas, making good mineral shortages by intelligent food supplementation, and by strict dietary control.

'It might also be necessary to make osteopathic or chiropractic adjustments. Compressed lesions in certain of the vertebrae can often be reflected in gastric and intestinal disturbances, producing toxins which the body may seek to eliminate via the skin.'

As already described, the tisanes or teas are made by adding boiling water to the herb, in the proportion of 1 oz (30g) of herb to 1 pint (570ml) of boiling water, drinking one small tea cup before meals, three times a day. Particularly during hot weather it is best to make a small quantity at a time, as otherwise the tea may deteriorate unless drunk within a day or two.

A combination which Thomas Bartram recommends is equal parts of nettles, centaury and red clover tops, all of which are beneficial to eczema. An old American favourite is saffron tea, which cleanses liver and kidneys, and other herbs which can be used in teas singly or together include burdock leaves, chamomile, dandelion leaves, figwort, plantain (major), clivers (or cleavers), ground ivy, chickweed, violet leaves and marigold flowers.

From the herbal pharmacy he recommends liquid extracts of *echinacea, arctium lappa, achillea millefolium, rumex crispus* and *smilax*, all taken with distilled water three times daily before meals.

Blue flag root, burdock root, sarsaparilla, poke root and sassafras root may also be prescribed in the form of a liquid extract, tincture or decoction (this is produced by boiling) but unless a preserve is added to the decoction it will not keep for more than three days.

Others find the most satisfactory way of taking herbs is in tablet form, and remedies readily available include many of the above plus chaparral, seaweed, golden seal and ginseng.

Creams and ointments

In Thomas Bartram's experience there is no one ointment that will relieve every case of eczema. 'Each person has to discover what suits them. But chickweed and comfrey have a considerable reputation, and many people use slippery elm and marshmallow ointment successfully. Some sufferers find an infusion of comfrey, chamomile, marshmallow or slippery elm helpful when bathed on to the affected areas.

'A comfrey poultice may succeed. Make this by placing three tablespoons of fresh or dried root in one pint of cold water, bring to the boil and simmer gently for fifteen minutes. Apply with a cloth, using three or four times a day when the eczema is dry.'

For dry eczema he also recommends jojoba cream, which assists the absorption of Vitamin A and moisturises and nourishes the skin's surface. Vitamin E in lotion or cream form, or a capsule punctured and smoothed over the skin is good, and so is evening primrose oil, used on the skin as well as taken internally.

Like other herbal practitioners, Thomas Bartram looks at the whole person when prescribing treatments, taking many aspects into consideration, including temperament, lifestyle, diet and possible allergies.

As a general guide to diet he recommends that one meal daily should consist of raw green vegetables only, with plenty of water to drink. He recommends plenty of apples, apricots, dates, figs, grapefruits, honey, lemons, peaches, prunes, beets, carrots, cauliflower, celery, lettuce, parsnips, radishes, sprouts, sweet potatoes, garlic, yogurt and kelp.

On the other hand he suggests rejecting red meats, anything from the pig (including bacon and ham), fried foods, sweets, pastries, white sugar and white flour products of all kinds, barbecue steaks, frankfurters. hamburgers, sausage, gravy powders, all cheese containing more than 1 per cent fat, cream and all cream substitutes, chocolate and carbonated drinks.

But much would depend on individual food sensitivities and intolerance, and diets such as those outlined in Chapter 6 might limit some of the fruits and other foods mentioned. As Thomas Bartram knows from his own experience, allergies can be wide-ranging and occasionally very surprising.

'Whether found in children or adults, eczema almost always has a strong family history and can be triggered off by a multitude of causes,' he says. 'With many people it may be due to allergy to proteins, but to many other things as well.

'A young agricultural student visited a pig house. Within three minutes she had a severe attack of asthma and it took an hour to recover her breath. Then her skin flared up with a fiery eczema.

'Drug-induced eczema is also common, and the nickel studs decorating a pair of jeans can be an overlooked cause in teenagers. There is even a variety of the disorder which attacks the face some days after striking matches. Allergy to phosphorus in a publican's wife became so troublesome that she did not lose her eczema until banning the sale of matches in her pub!'

Vitamins and supplements

Thomas Bartram recommends, like most herbalists, extra vitamins and supplements in the diet to make up for any deficiencies. But when discussing this need, you can find yourself in another chicken and egg situation. Does the deficiency lead to the eczema — or has the eczema led to certain deficiencies?

This can happen because the various diets used by children and adults with eczema may mean a lack of certain essential nutrients in the body. Even an apparently healthy vegan or vegetarian diet can result in a deficiency in vitamin B_{12} unless extra supplements are taken.

In a recent study at a children's hospital in Liverpool, twenty-three children on special diets, mostly excluding cow's milk and replacing it with a soya substitute, were tested for mineral intake, and the results compared with a control group of twenty-three children on a normal diet.

Thirteen of the children on special diets, but none among the control group, were found to have an intake of calcium less that 75 per cent of the normally recommended daily amount, and were also low in zinc. This made doctors feel that there were hazards involved in dieting which could make them dangerous unless a professional watch was kept on progress, particularly among children.

On the other hand, even those on what is regarded as a fairly normal diet nowadays may also be going short of certain important vitamins and minerals. Processed and convenience foods, and produce grown on poor soil which has been chemically treated, are likely to lack much of the goodness they once had.

So, regardless of special diets, there are many who would recommend the taking of special supplements each day to build up general health and resistance to illness, and also perhaps to mount a direct attack on the eczema itself.

As with so many other aspects of this condition, experience seems to vary as to which vitamins or supplements may be most helpful. A deficiency in Vitamin B_3, for instance, has been found by doctors to lead to rough skin. Vitamin D, manufactured by sunlight, regulates the amount of calcium and phosphorus in our bodies and has an important effect on growth and general health.

Vitamin E keeps cells healthy by ensuring a good blood-supply and helps heal sore skins and wounds. Vitamin F, found in many oils such as linseed, sunflower and evening primrose, helps our nails, complexion and skin conditions. Minerals such as zinc, calcium and selenium all play a part in healthy skin and body.

Two cases reported in *Exchange* show good results from the use of vitamin B_6. After reading an article in a health magazine, which said children with asthma had been helped by this particular supplement in their diet, one mother thought she would try it on her daughter.

'I started giving her 100mg of B_6 each morning and evening at the beginning of June as I knew that eczema and asthma are related and this vitamin can help allergies. By the beginning of August her eczema had disappeared, and also the slight hayfever my daughter had been suffering.

'She is still clear of eczema, but if I try to reduce the dosage the skin on her elbows becomes rough a few days later so I have decided to keep the 100mg night and morning all through the winter as the eczema always seems worse then. It is marvellous to see her legs without the ugly sore patches behind her knees.'

An adult who has had the same response says: 'I read in Adelle Davis' book *Let's Keep Fit* that vitamin B_6 was immediately helpful in cases of crusting and flaking skin. I started to take 30 mg a day, plus three soya lecithin capsules, and from that day my skin has steadily improved. I am so thankful — it is miraculous.'

Others have found multi-vitamin tablets, for instance capsules containing vitamins A, B, C and D have done the trick, or eating special foods rich in various nutrients such as brewer's yeast which includes the whole of the B group of vitamins apart from B_{12}, plus fourteen essential minerals.

Kelp, a type of seaweed, is rich in many minerals including calcium and potassium. Black molasses contain iron, and most of the B vitamins. Nutritious and tasty supplements essential to the macrobiotic diet are tahini, a sesame seed butter, and tamari and miso, both made from soya beans.

What is interesting is that many of these supplements and healthy foods seem able to feed the skin from the outside as well as the inside. People have had success from puncturing vitamin oil capsules and smoothing the contents onto the eczema rash and, as well as eating their yogurt and honey, have applied it to the skin.

Honey in particular appears to have many 'magical' ingredients, perhaps because of the active lives bees lead flitting from one health-giving herb and flower to another as they collect their pollen and make their combs. Even the 'cement' — called propolis — with which the bees seal the beehive is apparently good for you.

Healing oils

As we've already seen, oils of all sorts play a major part in easing eczema by lubricating and moisturizing the skin, sometimes working from the inside as well as the outside. It's almost as if the skin is being oiled from the inside out.

But equally important are the various supplements contained in the oils. One man who had had eczema all his life found that by taking eight to ten capsules of cod liver oil a day, his eczema has shown great improvement.

One mother gave her son four teaspoonfuls of pure corn oil a day and after a month his skin had become supple and smooth and she was able to stop using steroid preparations, though she still added emulsifying ointments to the bath. Another mother had similar success with her child by using sunflower oil.

Another oil which is having a marked affect on some cases of eczema is evening primrose oil, and part of the reason for this success is based on the theory that children with conditions such as eczema may be short of what are called essential fatty acids or polyunsaturates in the body.

Essential fatty acids are like most vitamins in that they cannot be made by the body but must be taken in via foods. The polyunsaturate of great importance in the human diet is called linoleic acid, contained in such vegetable oils as corn oil, sunflower and safflower.

The evening primrose is a wild flower growing mainly on the eastern coast of the U.S.A. and Canada, with seeds which produce an oil exceptionally rich in polyunsaturates and substantial amounts of something called 'gammalinolenic acid'.

In the body linoleic acid is normally converted into gammalinolenic acid, but a shortage of the essential fatty acid may prevent this happening. So the evening primrose oil short cuts the process, and makes up for any gammalinolenic acid deficiency.

As long ago as 1929 two Americans discovered that when linoleic acid was left out of the diet of animals, they developed eczema and hair loss, and it was claimed there was a link with children who had eczema. Various experiments were carried out adding maize oil and lard to the diet.

But after the coming of steroid treatments research was shelved, until a few years ago when various doctors became interested again, especially in the effects of evening primrose oil.

In particular one specialist, Dr John Burton of Bristol Royal Infirmary, carried out studies which showed the evening primrose oil capsules controlled the eczema of children and adults when used in sufficient quantities. Since then it has become the part of regular treatment for many people.

'I am fifty-seven and have had eczema all my life, so have tried and used every possible remedy,' says one woman. 'I heard about evening primrose oil capsules and have now been taking one 500mg capsule daily for exactly four months. I am quite sure that they have done me a lot of good.'

Writes a mother: 'I think our son, now aged eighteen, has been helped by taking B_6 and is now taking evening primrose oil capsules. He says the irritation has noticeably reduced and the condition of his skin has improved.'

More research is still going on into the remarkable properties of this oil, and at the time of writing this book manufacturers were hoping that it would soon be available on prescription as well as for sale across the chemist's counter.

Flower remedies

Another type of 'flower power' was discovered by a Dr Edward Bach in the 1930s. This Harley Street consultant and homoeopath gave up his London practice to devote his full time to seeking energies in the plant world which would restore vitality to the sick. The result of his work are the Bach Flower Remedies, still available today.

Yvonne Knibbs, who has used them along with homoeopathic remedies and diet to control her daughter's eczema, finds they help the whole family. The flowers are used not directly for physical complaints, but for negative states of mind and mood.

Says Yvonne: 'In the case of the eczema sufferer the state of mind may or may not be the initial cause but certainly it can be a contributing factor once the disease has manifested itself.

'It has been found that shock and trauma can have a long lasting effect on a person, and the Bach Flower Remedy is often prescribed for something that occurred years previously in order to cure the physical problems of the patient.'

In the end Dr Bach found thirty-eight flowers which he claimed covered all known negative states of mind from which mankind can suffer, categorizing them under seven headings — including apprehension, uncertainty and indecision, loneliness, insufficient interest in present circumstances, despondency and despair.

Says the Bach Flower Centre: 'They are a simple and natural method of establishing complete equilibrium and harmony through the personality, all prepared from the flowers of wild plants, bushes and trees, and none of them harmful or habit forming.

'As peace and harmony is achieved, unity returns to mind and body, closing the circuit and allowing the life force to flow freely again, thus providing the body its chance to produce its own natural healing.'

Healing Through

Homoeopathy

Judging from the letters I have received since starting this book, and also as editor of *Exchange*, homoeopathy seems to be among the most popular therapies for the treatment of eczema.

Perhaps some of its particular appeal for those new to holistic medicine is that it has a rather more medical feel to it than the rather off-beat therapies. In fact, some GPs are trained homoeopaths themselves and most appear to recognize homoeopathy as a legitimate form of medicine.

Whereas they might think twice about referring a patient to a dowser, herbalist or even acupuncturist, most seem to agree that homoeopathic methods could well hold the answers to some of the mysteries of a condition such as eczema.

Another reason for its popularity among natural therapies is that, perhaps even more than any others, homoeopathy takes the whole person into account before diagnosis is made and treatment prescribed. It isn't just symptoms and circumstances but sometimes the colour of hair and a patient's love of music that leads the practitioner to suggest one type of remedy rather than another.

It was in the eighteenth century that Dr Samuel Hahnemann, convinced that much orthodox medical practice did more harm than good, began to look for an alternative which would be safe, gentle and effective.

He believed that human beings have an innate capacity to heal themselves and reasoned that instead of suppressing symptoms he would seek to stimulate them and so encourage and assist the body's natural healing process.

Explains the Homoeopathic Development Foundation, one of several organizations involved in this field of medicine: 'Basing his work on the principal of "like curing like", Hahnemann found he could produce remedies by greatly diluting substances which in larger doses could have created symptoms similar to those seen in the patient.

'Hahnemann had already discovered that a small dose of quinine produced the symptoms of malaria in a healthy person. From this followed a number of systematic experiments and he found that remedies obtained from animal, vegetable, mineral and, more rarely biological, materials, were very effective in extreme dilutions, called potencies.

'Over a long period Hahnemann and his followers took small doses of various substances, carefully noting the symptoms they produced. These were called "provings". Subsequently, patients suffering from similar symptoms were treated with the substances.

'Hahnemann then worked to establish the smallest effective dose, for he realized that this was the best way to avoid side effects. In so doing, he also found that in general the more the remedy was diluted, the more effective it became.'

One of the principles of homoeopathy is that people will vary in their response to an illness according to their particular temperament, environment, family surroundings and medical history. For this reason the homoeopathic doctor will not automatically prescribe a specific remedy for a specific illness.

Because it is the patient who is being treated and not the disease, people with the same ailment may often need different remedies. On the other hand, another group of patients with different diseases could well benefit from the same remedy.

As one practitioner explains, reactions to all sorts of factors will be taken into consideration. Some people's symptoms are better in heat or cold, others are made worse by the type of weather, or are more severe during the night. These varying reactions are known as 'modalities'.

Giving an example of how these modalities can influence the choice of remedy, this practitioner mentions two homoeopathic medicines for treating rheumatism, *Causticum* and *Rhus Tox*. If the rheumatism is better in rainy weather then *Rhus Tox* might be recommended; if worse in rainy weather, then *Causticum* would probably be the answer.

Eczema and homoeopathy

Because of this very specific nature of diagnosis and treatments prescribed, it is very difficult for a practitioner to give any general guidelines on the treatment of eczema by homoeopathy.

Usually, changes in diet will be important, although again there is no officially laid down 'homoeopathic diet'. This will vary according to the individual and the picture of his or her life that the practitioner will build up through close questioning and perhaps a home visit.

Rest may be prescribed, and other changes in lifestyle that might result in less stress and anxiety, and a generally healthier mind and body. Other therapies such as osteopathy, acupuncture or mineral supplements might also be recommended.

During examination the good homoeopath will also use all modern aids of medical practice, taking blood-pressure, pulse rate, temperature and so on, and the results of these could lead to further suggestions.

But as far as the actual remedies prescribed, these will vary very much from person to person. As a specialist at the Royal Homoeopathic Hospital has explained: 'Very simply put, a remedy such as *Graphites,* in potency, is used for a wet eczema with a honey-like exudation in a child who is rather fat and tends to be constipated.

'On the other hand the remedy *Sulphur,* again in potency, is used when the picture presented is a burning, hot, dry skin always worse for the heat of the bed, with a tendency to infection in a patient who is thirsty, has an excellent appetite, who perspires easily and generally gives the unkempt appearance of Just William!'

With so many ifs and buts and sub-clauses involved, it isn't hard to see why you can't simply say that *Graphites* and *Sulphur* are recommended in the treatment of eczema even though these, along with *Mezareum, Psorinum* and *Rhus Tox* are among the remedies most frequently used. So in this chapter I rely mostly on patient experience on how homoeopathy has helped rather than giving a practitioner's blueprint for homoeopathic treatments.

For instance, the mother of 2-year-old Louise writes: 'Having no confidence in my local GPs and heartily sick of being told: "She will grow out of it in time — here is another tube of steroid cream," I felt weary and isolated. Help came when a health visitor advised me to go to the homoeopathic clinic in Manchester.

'What a refreshing change to be carefully listened to, copious notes taken, constructive advice given, but most important of all — a fresh approach. A strict diet was based on fresh vegetables, fruit, goat's milk, and yogurt and excluded fish, meat, and eggs, plus all foods containing additives and preservatives.

'Laura was also prescribed three doses of *Thuja*. The response to this treatment was amazing. Within a week her eczema had subsided and her temperament was considerably calmer and more rational. She has also received three doses of *Rhus Tox* and is at last sleeping through the night.'

Marilyn Harper took her young son Jeremy to a private homoeopath after finding that orthodox treatment with hydrocortisone was giving only temporary relief. After *Calc Carb* 30, three times a day for four days the cracks on his hands had gone and so had the eczema patches and dryness.

'He was given a repeat dose six months later. You can see occasional faint red patches below the surface of the skin, but they don't erupt or irritate, and seem to coincide with periods of teething. Our new GP is very sympathetic to homoeopathic treatments and impressed by Jeremy's results.'

The healing crisis

Jill Weigal had suffered from severe eczema on her hands plus excess use of steroid preparations for most of her twenty-six years when she came to homoeopathy. Her GP had suggested she use steroid creams under plastic gloves for increased absorption, a practice mostly frowned upon now since it also leads to an increase in side-effects.

'I was recommended to a medical practitioner who was also qualified in homoeopathy and was delighted to find that treatment consisted of lovely cooling, sweet smelling creams as well as various pills, potions and powders,' says Jill. 'I saw him often and regularly as he experimented to find out what suited me best.

'One unpleasant result of the change of treatment was an outbreak of infection with astonishingly painful boils coming up all over the place. I have read since this is not at all unusual when, after over-use, steroid creams are suddenly withheld, and for some time I had to stay in bed.'

But, with the combination of acupuncture, Jill has found that homoeopathic remedies do mostly keep her eczema at bay, and that whereas her hands were formerly hard, dry and wizened, they are now soft and supple in texture.

An example of an apparent miracle cure of a woman who had suffered from severe eczema for over forty-two years appeared in the magazine *Exchange*. But she, too, had to suffer a period of feeling worse before feeling better.

Writes her husband, 'She was undergoing the most dramatic healing process, shedding layer after layer of skin, but all the time we were sustained by the fact that the practitioner told us what was going to happen.

'When using homoeopathic treatment there are times when the practitioner expects the patient will go through a healing crisis, and at times like these it is essential that the patient has complete rest. The patient will feel very low and complete rest will hasten the process, whereas to try to carry on a normal daily life will make the crisis much longer.'

Twelve months later this lady's skin was better than at any time in her life, beautifully soft and smooth according to her husband. On top of this her general health problems, some due to long-term use of steroids, had been sorted out, too.

'The cure can be called miraculous, but in my belief it is due to a doctor who above all cares for her patients and who by using her powers of observation sets out to treat the cause of the illness rather than trying to suppress the symptoms,' comments Jill's husband.

A mother whose daughter was treated by a homoeopathic doctor found it was this aspect of care and interest that was most valuable. She felt she and her husband were helped to understand their daughter as well as her physical ailment and benefitted from what she describes as 'an enormous amount of emotional support.'

Unhappy choice

Unfortunately not everyone is so lucky, and I feel it is important to include the experience of one adult patient, Cheryl Gordon, who writes to say that in her case a course of homoeopathy resulted in near breakdown.

Because her eczema developed for the first time when she was already twenty-one years old, most experienced doctors would look first to see whether she was suffering from the contact type of eczema, caused by some factor in her life that was acting as an irritant or allergen.

Instead, the homoeopath Cheryl visited prescribed various pills after which the eczema became very much worse and stayed that way for almost a year. Because she had been warned about the healing crisis, Cheryl stuck it out without resorting to antibiotics, even though her eczema was now badly infected, but her worried husband did summon the homoeopath back.

'She arrived with a small computer which she plugged into our televison and with no further ado, without chatting to me about my problems, typed in each and every one of my symptoms,' remembers Cheryl. 'The word sulphur appeared on the screen, apparently showing that this was the treatment to be used for my exact condition.

'She leant back in her chair and sighed, stating: "The computer says I'm giving you the right remedies, so really it should have worked." She then handed me more pills to take every day to calm me down for a week, and suggested that I then see her colleague for a second opinion.

'I was devastated. I had been led to believe that homoeopathic treatment was given according to personal circumstances, habits, personality, likes and dislikes of the individual, and the remedies were given in varying amounts depending on that individual. I was horrified to realise that a computer programme was treating me and not the therapist.'

In the event, Cheryl needed a week in hospital to recover and now wonders whether she would have done better to have gone to a GP who practised homoeopathy rather than a therapist, because then perhaps there would have been more likelihood of action being taken sooner when the infection developed.

But perhaps the more important lesson to be learned from this is to choose a practitioner with care, preferably recommended personally. Homoeopathy, like other therapies, has its charlatans, and it is essential to check credentials before undertaking treatment.

Taking the medicine
A few other points are worth bearing in mind when judging the success

or otherwise of homoeopathic treatment. It may puzzle some patients how such a tiny dose can have any effect at all. But it is the frequency at which the dose is taken that is important, and sometimes this will be every three or four hours.

As one practitioner explains, from experience homoeopaths have found that low potencies (i.e., those in which dilution has not been carried out) are short-lasting and superficial in effect. Medium potencies are longer-acting and can influence a wider and deeper range of symptoms, while the high potencies (i.e., those in which there is most dilution) are more fundamental still in their effects.

These are best prescribed by the homoeopath, and self-help treatments which can be bought through homoeopathic chemists should only be in the low potency range.

Another general rule mentioned by this practitioner is that, unless changes in condition are noticed in the first twenty-four hours (and remember these may sometimes be for the worse as well as the better) it is very likely that the choice of remedy is incorrect. But all this should be carried out under the advice and watchful eye of a qualified homoeopath.

Once sufficient progress has been made, the homoeopath would reduce the dosage or even stop it altogether. But this will not necessarily mean that treatment is over. The remedies can go on working in the body long after they are taken, one of the basic beliefs of homoeopathy being that the medicines stimulate the body's own healing powers.

Mineral supplements
As we've already seen, mineral deficiencies in the body are thought to contribute towards eczema, and this is another area where homoeopathic treatment can be very helpful.

One way of supplementing minerals in the diet, and a safe self-help treatment, is with the use of biochemic tissue salts. There are twelve basic salts, plus eighteen combinations, each one suited to particular ailments or symptoms.

Nano Donoghue, who had been struggling unsuccessfully with her young daughter's eczema since she was a baby of six weeks, met a woman who was treating her little boy with tissue salts. Remembers Nano:

'I was sceptical — you become so after many failures — but curious, so I bought a biochemic handbook from the local health store. The book told me that a tissue salt named *calcium fluoride* was beneficial for cracks in the palms or hands so I bought some.

'I actually have Claire on four salts at the moment, each acting on problems associated with eczema — thickening of skin, lack of perspiration, skin slow to heal, and on the eczema itself. Her skin is now a lot better. Not cured, but she no longer has the cracks and loves her baths. Best of all, she is a lot happier.'

The mother of a five-year-old daughter writes how, following a bout of eczema herpeticum and then measles, her daughter's skin was in a dreadful state. She had already tried elimination diets and every prescribed cream on the market, all to no avail. So she went to see a homoeopath who specialized in mineral therapy.

'He took a cutting of her hair for analysis, examined her eyes, mouth and skin and diagnosed a mineral deficiency. She was put on a course of minerals which at first seemed to slightly aggravate the condition but then the miracle happened and her eczema started to disappear.

'The minerals prescribed were *potassium sulphate* and *magnesium phosphate, sodium phosphate, silica* and *calcium fluoride*, all in tablet form taken several times a day. She was also prescribed iron at at first, but that is no longer needed.

'Her appetite returned, she had improved energy and the condition of her hair and nails improved. I was also told to give her less sugar and no citrus fruits. I have always given her four evening primrose oil capsules daily, which also seems to help.'

Osteopath Jeanette Thomson also uses mineral compounds for treating eczema as a part of what is called cellular therapy. This stems from the work of an Australian, Maurice Blackmore. 'He was a naturopath who devised a method which employed the use of mineral compounds in doses which could be assimilated by the body,' explains Jeanette.

'These mineral compounds are only ten in number and the patient is treated according to the totality of his or her symptoms and signs, as in homoeopathy.

'This system recognizes mineral deficiencies to be the common denominator of most illnesses, and these compound minerals are in no way disruptive to the body's mineral reserves. I use this therapy on a number of patients in conjunction with osteopathy and diet, and have seen excellent results.'

It's worth bearing in mind, by the way, that illness can result from an excess of certain minerals in the body as well as deficiency. Lead poisoning through air pollution, piping or paints is a typical example.

Though it is possible to have blood tests through your local hospital to test an iron deficiency, for instance, you can also have hair analysed to show up any mineral imbalance. An address to contact can be found in the reference section at the back of the book.

In Touch with Energy

Acupuncture and some of its allied therapies remain mysterious to many people. Unlike herbalism, homoeopathy and naturopathy, which have a fairly practical application to our lives, acupuncture with its talk of energy flow and life forces seems more other-worldly and intangible.

Yet all of us recognize these forces in our lives in the ebb and flow of feeling and moods, and the strong attractions and repulsions we experience towards certain things, places or people.

We talk of having 'no energy' when we feel ill, tired or depressed. Yet when we are happy and in good spirits we can feel ourselves bursting with exuberance and life — in other words, full of energy.

That these feelings affect our health as well is also obvious, though perhaps we are more inclined to blame a feeling of being generally out of sorts and at odds with the world on a headache or upset stomach, rather than the other way round.

For thousand of years, oriental medical practitioners have been aware of these energy patterns that relate to the various body functions. They believe that the body is run by energy which, in the healthy person, is perfectly distributed within all the systems of the body.

But when these energies are disturbed in some way through stress, whether physical, chemical or psychological, then the functions of the whole body are thrown out of balance, leading eventually to ill health.

So the aim of the many oriental-based therapies is to detect this imbalance and then to put it right, so that the energies are unblocked and can flow freely again, and the body will therefore be balanced and more healthy.

Acupuncture

As always, the proof is in the results and there seems no doubt that however mysterious it may be, therapies like acupuncture *do* work and many people have been healed by them.

This is really how acupuncture came to be discovered in the first place. As the British Acupuncture Association describes in an introductory booklet, many thousands of years ago it was noted in China that soldiers wounded by arrows sometimes recovered from illnesses which had afflicted them for years. The Chinese then began to copy the effects of the arrow by artificially puncturing the skin.

'The theory behind acupuncture,' explains the Association, 'is that there exists in the body dual flows of energy called Yin and Yang, containing within them an overall conception of energy known as Chi, or life force.

'These are expressed in everything in the universe — day and night, elasticity and contractability, hot and cold, life and death. Everything has its force of opposition, but this opposition by its very existence is itself complementary.

'Yang tends to stimulate, to contract, and is the positive principle, while Yin tends to sedate, to expand, and is the negative principle. Health is dependent on the equilibrum of Yin and Yang, firstly within the body and secondly within the entire universe.'

The Chinese believe that this vital energy circulates in the body along the meridians, similar to the blood, nerve and lymphatic circuits. Interestingly, the flow along the meridians may be detected in the living body by electronic and other means, but it disappears at death.

The body keeps Yin and Yang in harmony by dispelling surplus energy via the skin's surface at various points. Traditionally there are about 800 of these points, but new ones are continually being discovered. When the energy flow is unbalanced and symptoms of illness appear, then the skin is pierced at points relevant to these symptoms, and to the individual concerned.

As one practitioner explains, the cause of the pain or illness may lie at a considerable distance from the visible or felt malfunction. He likens it to the electric light that won't work — first we would check the bulb, secondly the light switch, then the light fuse, then the main fuse.

So it is, he says, with the body's energy currents. The acupuncturist can follow the meridian until he or she finds the fault and corrects it. But obviously, over years of practice, they have built up a wealth of experience as to which points need activating for a certain set of symptoms.

Most acupuncture is carried out by traditional methods, but even ancient arts move with the times and there is now a method of electro-acupuncture which actually assesses the states of Yin and Yang energy flows, and can treat accordingly.

Moxibustion is a form of acupuncture using heat, and in ear acupuncture small needles are applied only to the ears, different areas of which correspond with various parts of the unborn foetus.

The acupuncturist believes that there must be a balance of energy in the patient's environment as well as in the body and the philosophy embraces exercise, the food that is eaten, the water that is drunk and the air that is breathed. Ideally, everything in life should be balanced and in harmony.

Acupuncture and eczema

Peter Smith is an osteopath and acupuncturist who has treated patients with eczema. In his experience the imbalances of energy leading to conditions like this are caused by faulty diet, climatic conditions, shock or extremes of emotion, including joy as well as grief and anger.

He also believes that either diet or acupuncture used alone are limited in the treatment of eczema, and need to be used together for success. He recommends a wholefood diet excluding every possible allergen, plus relaxation, massage, manipulation, herbalism, and consideration of the patient's emotional state and external environment.

One of his patients was a boy of eleven suffering from eczema and asthma. There were many flare-ups when the skin became cracked and weeping, and steroid creams had been used daily, often with antibiotics.

'The family had tried to reduce the steroid creams many times with no success,' Peter Smith reports. 'In the first two months of treatment there were several flare-ups which he managed to get through without resorting to antibiotics. The steroid cream was slowly withdrawn over this period.

'To date, four years later, there have been no flare-ups, and the general condition of the skin is much improved though ankles and wrists remain very dry. But there has been no recurrence of the asthma since the first treatment.'

'Another patient was a boy of seventeen with eczema so severe that physical and psychological suffering had led him to consider suicide. He was treated weekly for four months, over which time the steroid cream was slowly withdrawn. There was a dramatic improvement both in the eczema and his psychological state.'

But in the case of a boy of seven, treatment with needles became too much of an ordeal and had to be stopped. Acupressure without needles was also tried, but was not helpful. This highlights the problem of acupuncture needling for young children, as in Peter Smith's experience the two rarely mix. But the story of one mother who has contacted me, Debra Webster, shows that this is not always so.

Her son Saul was born with a very dry skin, and eczema developed soon after, although she was breast-feeding. Even on a cow's milk-free and egg-free diet, plus hydrocortisone from the GP, he did not improve.

Her final disillusionment with orthodox methods of controlling the eczema came when a skin specialist prescribed an even stronger hydrocortisone, looked at her as if she was mad when she said that Saul drank no cow's milk and suggested it was an old wives' tale that dairy products were harmful.

'I came away from him vowing never to go back,' Debra remembers. 'I was recommended to an acupuncturist specializing in treating children, but at first was reluctant to go. Then five weeks ago I took Saul and was amazed at the result.

'He was treated with one needle in four places — his wrists, and just above his knees. The needle was very fine and the acupuncturist applied surgical spirit first. He also gave me a solution of herbs for Saul to take daily, and recommended applying *Calendula* cream.

'Since then Saul has had the needle in six points, as before and on his foot at the bottom of each big toe. Saul screamed when the needles first went in but I think that was more because someone was doing something to him than because it hurt. Afterwards he was given some raisins, and became quiet again immediately.

'He now looks like any other two-year-old and I have cut down his medicine by about half and he still sleeps through the night. He is calmer than ever before. The acupuncturist says that he is treating his digestive system which is the root of his illness and that it will also calm him down. This is certainly what has happened and I have changed from a definite disbeliever to a complete follower.

'Saul certainly does not enjoy it but we go once a week and he does not get unduly upset even though he knows where we are going. It is not only me or the immediate family but outsiders as well who have remarked on the improvement in Saul's temper and skin. I am delighted and would recommend it to anyone.'

Do it yourself

Although the application of needles would be dangerous in the hands of an untrained person, there are forms of acupressure and other therapies which use the same energy principles for self-help treatment.

For instance, bone needles which do not penetrate the skin can be held on the acupuncture points, unblocking or releasing energy in the same way as needles. As an acupunturist who uses this method explains, it is not so much the instrument that is important, but the correct location of the relevant points.

He suggests buying a handbook, looking up eczema or other symptoms allied to the condition, finding the correct pressure points on the body from the diagrams supplied, and then applying the bone massager.

'Similar meridians run through both sides of the body so if you have to action a point on the left foot, you should also action the similar point on the right foot,' he says.

'To find the right point can take time and experience, but there are clues. If the point needs actioning, it will be tender to the touch. When sure of the point and using massage you will get one of the following sensations — a pin prick, a sharp needle, a red hot burning sensation or a warm glow.

'Hold the massager on the point until the sensation disappears. If there are any pricking sensations in other parts of the body during this time, move the massager to that point next time and repeat the process.'

This practitioner also suggests that, as far as possible, eczema sufferers who are using acupuncture of any sort try and avoid scratching itchy spots of the body, as these may be acupuncture points needing action. Instead, place the point of the bone needle on the spot and see what happens!

'Some acupuncturists will tell you that the particular meridians have to be actioned at certain times of the day. Whilst this is true, it holds no problems in self-healing. The times for actioning the points coincides with those times when the illness is at its most distressing, in other words when you feel the need for relief the most.'

Shiatsu

Shiatsu is a Japanese word meaning 'finger pressure' and it is like acupuncture but this time instead of needles the hands and body pressure are used. There are also different styles of Shiatsu, some concentrating on pressure points and others covering wider areas of the meridians.

As with all these therapies, the aim of Shiatsu is to balance energy by the application of touch and pressure. The practitioner uses his body as a kind of channel for energy and because hands are involved there is also a healing quality to it.

Practitioners find it particularly suitable for conditions such as eczema which can be made worse by stress or anxiety, and in fact the whole approach is towards mental as well as physical relaxation.

Shiatsu is practised on mats on the floor and both the patient and the therapist wear loose clothes. The whole body is treated, although more attention is paid to any problem areas and diagnosis and treatment are part of the same process. Breathing is important, and pressure is applied with each outbreath. Massage is used first to loosen up the muscles, and then pressure applied to the appropriate points.

Shiatsu can be learned by anyone and some clinics hold practice groups. There is also a type of do-it-yourself Shiatsu called Do-in (pronounced doe-in). This consists of a series of exercises, mostly carried out sitting down, starting in the 'Seisa' position, kneeling with the hands folded in the lap.

There is a brief preparation co-ordinating the breathing with bending to the ground and then a sequence of movements dealing in order with the hands, wrists, arms, head, chest, shoulders, waist, legs, feet, pelvis, abdomen and back.

Each stage involves a combination of moving the hands over the body, first without touching, then massaging along the meridians in the direction of the energy flow, then with vigorous massage of muscles and joints (where energy can apparently get stuck) and finally with pressure applied to the points using the pad of the thumb.

Again, this therapy helps towards peace of mind as well as health of body. It is preventative as well as curative, ideally aiming to stop illness developing in the first place.

Reflexology

Once grasped, the whole concept of energy patterns and rhythms in the body starts to make sense of other therapies. Reflexology, which involves massage and pressure to the feet, I had always thought of as a particularly obscure and unlikely method of healing, but now can see how it fits into the general picture.

Like other 'zone therapies', as they are called, it is based on the theory that as the body's systems all have terminal points in the extremities — feet, hands, skull and so on — pressure applied there can clear up malfunction in specific nerves, organs or glands.

Like so many natural therapies, reflexology is very ancient and, according to the International Institute of Reflexology, was used in Egypt as far back as 2330 B.C. It is still very popular in Eastern countries, and moved to the Western world with a lady physiotherapist in Florida who became very interested in its benefits.

The Institute holds regular training meetings and a professional training course, and has a register of qualified reflexologists. One practitioner who has treated people with eczema among his patients is Roger Locke.

He admits that it is not known precisely how zone therapy in general and reflexology in particular work, but they are thought to operate on the nervous system through 'switching points' on the spine which link different segments of the body.

'It's also thought you get a crystalline deposit on the nerve endings where these or glands are under stress of some sort. When you press the finger or thumb on some points it feels as though a needle is going in.

'Obviously, massage helps to remove waste deposits from the feet, clearing congestion and blockages from energy pathways and balancing negative and positive. It normalizes glands and organ functioning, and relaxes mind and body.'

The patient removes shoes and socks and sits in a comfortable chair with his or her feet up — a nice experience in itself! The feet are then massaged gently before beginning pressure on the various appropriate points.

'Reflexology is very accurate diagnostically,' says Roger Locke, 'as, when you are giving treatment, you are diagnosing at the same time. The therapy will throw up conditions that a person has had in the past as well as present conditions and possible future problems.'

He has had several successes with both adults and children with eczema, though he points out this is not always the case. One twelve-year-old girl who suffered from eczema and asthma cleared after nine months of treatment, and a woman with contact eczema, who was allergic to nickel, lost the rash on her hands after two sessions, but continued treatment for some time to keep up the goods results.

'It is necessary to persevere with the treatment,' says Roger Locke. 'Normally, treatment will need to go on for many months, sometimes years, to receive full benefit. It may also be necessary to make adjustments in the diet, to avoid certain allergens — such as nickel — and to have mineral and vitamin supplements.'

Touch for Health
Touch for Health is a modern off-shoot of a very ancient therapy, kinesiology. In both, the muscles are used to test the energy lines and levels of the body, and to put right any imbalances or disharmonies that are found.

The therapist tests muscle tone, not its strength or weakness in the sense of being able to pick up enormous weights or flex bulging arms and legs. To judge tone, the therapist positions the limbs in turn and then applies pressure in a certain direction, asking the patient to resist.

Once this has been done, various techniques are used to subdue the muscles that have too much energy and stimulate those that don't have enough. For instance, pain is often a sign of too much concentrated energy and this can be put right by gently applying pressure to other muscles to balance the tension. Local massage of the meridians and pressure points may also be included in treatment.

The Touch for Health organization explains in an introductory leaflet that these simple muscle tests can detect imbalances in the circulatory, neuromuscular and meridian energy systems of the body, and can also find out about dietary deficiencies and unfavourable reactions to food and drink.

'In using Touch for Health muscle tests we are really asking the body itself to tell us about its problems and needs. With the first-hand knowledge thus gained we can apply the simple yet powerful therapies to restore balance, increase energy, improve posture, relieve pain, depression and stress, and promote general well-being.

'While it is not a cure-all and does not replace professional care, Touch for Health is a wonderful way of improving your own health and that of family and friends. It is easy to learn and safe and simple to apply, and can be used by the layperson with no previous experience as well as being a useful additional skill of the professional therapist. It is, in fact, being learned and used by many chiropractors and osteopaths.'

12.

Mind and Body

Almost all the natural therapies discussed so far have touched on the mental and emotional influences on the physical, and the need for wholeness and harmony in mind, body and spirit.

To be tense, unhappy and anxious does affect the correct functioning of every part of the body, and it seems logical that this can lead to a general feeling of not being well, and eventually to specific symptoms and illness.

Not, I would repeat, that I and many others I have talked to, would support the over-simplistic theory that eczema and other skin conditions are 'all due to nerves'. As we've already seen, it is understandable that the person who has a disfiguring rash and never-ending agony of itching, not to mention the social problems that can arise from this, will become irritable and depressed at times.

But this is often more a result of the illness, rather than the cause of it. Though not generally thought of as a serious handicap in physical terms, eczema has nevertheless crippled some people's lives because of its effects, and in some instances led to suicide.

As one young woman, Johanna Fawkes, wrote in a *Guardian* article: 'It is no surprise that eczema leads to hyperactivity, tension, anger, frustration, despair and loneliness. Most sufferers have to deal with constant itching, overheating, bleeding and soreness.

'A smile or a short walk can be painful, swimming or playing games is out of the question. It leads to rejection by other children at school, and insinuations of blame in adulthood. No wonder peace and harmony occasionally give way to anger.'

Johanna describes years of thinking that really her eczema was all in her mind, and that if she weren't so neurotic it would go away. Like many others she had misunderstood the word psychosomatic — which means the action of mind on body — for psychological — which means 'in the mind'.

'Over the years I have absorbed all the half-informed remarks of teachers, doctors and others who hear the word psychosomatic and equate it with something that can be controlled at will,' she goes on. 'If you want to stop the pain enough you can do it. Failure indicates lack of resolution and self-destructive tendencies.'

Johanna then describes the great relief she felt when she learned from more knowledgeable people the real facts about her illness, which was triggered by a mixture of things, including heredity, acute sensitivity to certain substances, and allergy.

But even though the prime cause of eczema may not be nervous or emotional, like any other disorder from stomach ulcers to cancer, it can be made worse by tensions and conflicts in the mind which will attack the body's most vulnerable point.

In the case of the person with an already weak heart, stress might lead to a heart attack. In those who have a weak digestion the outcome could be colitis, and in those with breathing or lung problems it could be asthma.

In the person who because of hereditary and immunological disorders, and other reasons not yet discovered, is predisposed to skin disorders, then the result could be eczema. So though in the same family there might be a brother and sister experiencing exactly the same atmosphere and tensions, one will develop eczema and the other won't.

Because of this it is obviously a helpful step to work towards greater peace of mind and relaxation of body. We all have to live with stress in this world, but at least we can find ways of coping better with it.

This doesn't have to be a lonely battle, with a feeling of guilt and self-blame attached to it. Instead it can be seen as just a part of the whole health picture, and a goal for which most people, whether or not they have eczema, are aiming nowadays.

What is encouraging, too, is that there is a great deal of help available if you know where to look. In the end it may only be ourselves who can change our own way of thinking and living, but at least there are many people around to guide us on the way.

Talking it through

What most of us need more than anything in the world is the chance to talk about the problems connected with eczema. Parents crave the opportunity to pour their hearts out to someone about their weariness at coping with broken nights, blood-stained clothing and a scratching child, their frustrations at failed treatments, their guilt that their child has eczema at all.

Adults patients equally need to let go of their resentment and frustration. 'Why me?' so many ask. 'Why should it be me who has to live with a sore and sometimes unsightly skin, the stares of other people, the unkind comments, the daily toil of putting on creams and taking baths?'

I remember when my son was still quite young having a dream in which our usually cold and distant skin specialist suddenly turned towards me with a warm, sympathetic smile and said: 'Now Christine, tell me how things are.' The relief I felt that he actually wanted to hear was so great I can still remember it.

Unfortunately that was a dream, and all too often specialists and doctors either do not have the time or the inclination to talk about the emotional and social difficulties connected with eczema. They will briefly discuss creams and antihistamines and maybe touch on allergy, but there isn't often an opportunity for family or patient to discuss the real problems.

Unfortunately, if doctors are interested in the psychological side of things, it is all too often to blame the condition on to this rather than see it as part of the complex set of factors that it is. Mother and father are too tense/protective/uncaring; child is dominated/manipulative/unloved; adult patient is self-effacing/over aggressive/anxious — the result, according to some, is eczema.

One of our worst experiences as a family was with a skin specialist who obviously prided himself on being an amateur pyschologist. When Adam went into his hospital we were initially told we could not visit him at all — and he was then eight years old.

Later my husband and I were subjected to Nazi-type interrogation, and his eczema blamed on every conceivable aspect of our lives, from the fact that we have moved house a few times to the accusation that we had never really loved him.

The result of this was months of anguish and guilt, which made it even more difficult to cope calmly and rationally with our son's problems. Help came in the form of another skin specialist who, when he heard about our experience, confided that this man was an extremist, and his views not to be taken seriously. Again, the relief was enormous.

Unbottling feelings

So, somewhere in between lies the real help, with a person who acknowledges that dealing with the emotional and mental aspects and resulting social problems is an important part of treating eczema, but only a part of a multi-faceted picture.

Says Dennis Brown, a psychologist who has talked with many eczema patients: 'My views are that eczema is a particular skin reaction which takes many different clinical forms and frequently appears in transient episodes (like my own).

'It can be provoked and kept going by a number of physical factors such as external irritants, allergies and infections, and predisposed to in some by genetic factors. This is not a new idea. As long ago as 1842 the great dermatologist Erasmus Wilson included what he called "affections of the nervous system, particularly of the depressing kind" among causes of eczema, along with skin irritants, season, climate, irritating food and drink and digestive disorders.

'Inevitably, just as types of eczema differ, so do patients. Their temperaments and ways of dealing with problems and feelings vary as widely as any other group of people. But incomplete expression of feelings can contribute to the causation and perpetuation of eczema — particularly feelings of frustration, resentment and depression.'

So what is really needed is the chance to vent our feelings, maybe on the chatty level of one mother sympathizing with another over the piles of washing, but more often in a deeper vein so that the pent-up emotions Dr Brown refers to can come out.

In ordinary day-to-day life this isn't always easy to do, particularly when you are trying to create a happy and peaceful atmosphere in the home for a child with eczema, or attempting to lead an ordinary life with working colleagues or friends. Writes one young woman of twenty-seven:

'One of the best pieces of advice ever given to me was by a woman who told me (when I was at the tender age of sixteen and going through all the agony of developing and becoming aware of my appearance and finding it severely lacking) that I should always let my feelings be shown.

' "Shout, scream, rant and rave but never bottle up your feelings, it makes the condition much worse, somehow," she said. For me her advice was relevant, and I've remembered her words and tried to follow them, even at the risk of making workmates and friends think I'm highly strung or a bit dotty!'

Parents will have the same need to show their feelings as they watch a child tearing at his or her skin, or limping off sadly to school. But because it is important not to transfer anxiety to the child, much of the release must be done in private.

'If I felt het up then I'd leave the room,' says one mother whose daughter with eczema is now adult. 'I might go and bang my head against the wall in sheer frustration at times, but I'd do it somewhere on my own and never in front of my daughter.'

One specialist speaks of the need for parents to be very good at acting, and also to accept the child's eczema, just as teenage or adult patients should try and accept theirs. '"Love me, love my itch. Accept me, accept my itch" should be the message,' he says.

It's also vital to accept that there will be good and bad phases and not feel guilty about it. As he points out, this is a natural part of eczema and no-one's fault.

Counselling therapy

This consultant happens to be one who for many years held group meetings with his patients where they could talk through their worries and compare their feelings and reactions with other people, often with very good results.

Exploring your deeper emotions like this can sometimes give you a different and more positive perspective. In one hospital the medical social worker arranged group discussions for some of the teenagers with eczema attending the outpatients' department.

He discovered that though, on occasion, these young people had genuine grievances over attitudes of teachers at school, teasing from their peers and nagging at home, because of these experiences and the teenagers' rather negative feelings about themselves, they did tend to read rejection and criticism into the slightest remark or look.

By discussion and comparison they began to realize this could be true, and also by sharing their problems and feeling less alone could face up better to unpleasant situations when they did arise. The right word or response, a simple explanation of what eczema really is, can very quickly put ignorant or unthinking people in their place.

With the wisdom of hindsight my son can now see that most of the people who hurt him so much as a child were, in fact, not worth bothering about anyway because they were usually the bullies, or sad people with worse problems of their own.

Another way of gaining this new outlook and release is through the various self-awareness and therapy groups that exist in most towns and cities now. Once known as 'encounter' groups and tarred with a rather suspect reputation for baring the body as well as the soul, there are now many that give sound help and support to all sorts of people.

The usual pattern is to discuss individual problems in the presence of a facilitator who can guide discussion and give professional support. Other members of the group will also be encouraged to show understanding, both verbally and physically, with hugs and cuddles.

Some groups use techniques such as pyschotherapy, when different members take on particular roles in a group member's life — i.e. the child with eczema, the worried parent, the doctor who simply won't understand. Then particularly troublesome experiences can be acted out and perhaps resolved.

Or maybe a cushion will take the place of that awkward doctor or difficult child, or even the eczema itself, and the person will be encouraged to shout and punch the negative feelings out.

Individual and family therapy with a trained psychologist or psychiatrist can also be necessary and helpful if tensions and disturbance have reached a high level. This may be arranged through the skin department of a hospital, or can be found through an organization such as the Tavistock Clinic in London.

It was by going to family therapy that one mother realized how much her younger daughter's eczema was affecting the whole family and its peace of mind. Sitting and talking together they found they could all begin to see each other's point of view.

'I had always boasted how understanding my elder daughter had been about bedtime routines,' says the mother. 'Whereas I spent half an hour or so with the little one, applying ointments and soothing her, sometimes holding her hands and trying to talk her to sleep, I would then pop into the older one, kiss her goodnight and go downstairs. She never complained.

'Obviously there were many times when the younger daughter needed a great deal of attention. But the therapy sessions showed me that my older child was jealous and even resented me. So I had to try and help the older girl as well as the younger.'

Hypnotherapy and eczema

Hypnosis is often used as a part of psychotherapy nowadays, and is then called hypnotherapy. It is a different thing altogether from hypnosis as entertainment, when the hypnotist fixes staring eyes upon his clients, persuading them to do all sorts of weird and wonderful things.

Instead, a professionally-trained hypnotherapist will use the technique to reach the deeper parts of the mind more easily. This way hidden problems may be revealed, and certain ideas accepted which may improve a condition such as eczema, or at least make it easier to deal with.

A positive rather than negative circle can be set up so that, by feeling more relaxed about the condition, the sufferer may improve, and having improved physically will then feel even better mentally and emotionally.

Methods used will vary a lot from therapist to therapist. Often, the even level of a voice, the repetition of certain words, or the movements of a pen or pendulum will be sufficient to send the patient off into the state of deep relaxation and concentration which is hypnosis.

Many believe this to be like sleep, but in fact people under hypnosis are often more aware than usual and can keep their eyes open, speak, and remember what happened afterwards. But the altered state of consciousness can lead to profound relaxation, deeper breathing and the recollection of apparently forgotten incidents.

Qualified therapists are often members of the British Hypnotherapy Association which claims many victories for eczema sufferers and has a register of members. Another organization is the British Society of Medical and Dental Hypnosis who can also put patients in touch with suitable practitioners. Addresses are in the reference section at the end of this book.

One orthodox skin specialist uses hypnosis as part of his work. On the whole he does not see this as a cure, but rather as a way of suggesting to the person under hypnosis that things are getting better.

'One method of help can be by direct symptom removal to stop the itch,' he explains. 'However, I rarely have this as my sole directive when treating patients. The effect of the disease process is not only due to the condition itself, but also to the interaction of the individual.

'Particular emotions can bring about exacerberations, for example emotional stress in eczema. My particular aims with hypnosis are therefore to lessen the destructive emotional problems, and to help the patient cope with particular stresses which may provoke it.'

That hypnosis can help is borne out by the story of Hilary Smith, a teenager whose severe eczema had caused her many problems in education and employment. She was out of work, depressed and overdependent on home and parents, and the whole family was at the end of their tether.

Having been told by their skin specialist that there was nothing more to be done, Hilary went to a hypnotist who was also a medical practitioner. Treatment consisted of several visits to him for hypnosis, plus a good deal of talking.

'It was like a miracle', reported Hilary's mother. 'Two months later she had moved into her own flat and two months after that she had a job as a nursery assistant at a hospital for mentally and physically handicapped.

'Throughout the year we have seen improvement from a hunched weakling to a fit, healthy girl full of life with no eczema, a job she loves and a home of her own — and what is more she can eat anything.'

Not everyone has quite such a positive experience. Our son, for instance, showed no improvement in his eczema after several fairly costly hypnosis sessions. But rather, as at the faith healing services we once attended, he enjoyed the relaxing sensations and certainly the experience did no harm.

Faith healing

Many people turn to spiritual healing in their search for some way to ease the eczema. One lady even wrote to *Exchange* to say that keeping a copy of the twenty-third psalm tucked into her stocking tops had kept her rash at bay!

Another wrote to say that, having tried acupuncture, herbal remedies and hypnotherapy with no success, spiritual healing had made her skin calmer and less inflamed for the first time in years.

The Aetherius Society believes in spiritual healing in conjunction with all natural therapies, using what they call the prana or Universal Life Force which they believe is all around us. They also carry out absent healing, when hundreds of miles can separate healer and patient, and self healing.

Maureen Butler found that Christian healing helped her young daugher. 'Christian healing is concerned with the whole person, physical, mental and spiritual,' she says. 'Also it is not a magic cure — people are not always healed instantly. Some may not be physically healed at all, but they find the strength to cope with their situation.

'Mary Anne was prayed for by lots of people over a period of time. She also had hands layed on and when she was very bad we had a healing service in our home when she was prayed for and anointed with oil.

'She was healed mentally and spiritually and the eczema is improving all the time. She has changed from being a nervous, introvert child into a very happy and confident one. I am sure that the best treatments for eczema are the ones that seek to heal the whole person.'

Massage and relaxation

As we've already seen, touch and massage can have a healing effect on the body for quite physical reasons. But they can also relax and comfort the mind and spirit in a way which is very beneficial to health.

There are various forms of massage therapy, including aromatherapy, in which oils are used which match the patient's personality, and this in itself could have a healing effect on the skin.

There is also Swedish massage which uses several techniques, including manipulation of the muscle tissue and friction, to increase blood circulation, stimulate glands in the skin, soothe and rest bodies and ease pain.

Yoga, relaxation classes and meditation are all helpful to people with eczema, not just because they relax both physically and mentally but because they also encourage a feeling of control over one's own body and destiny.

Yoga is a particularly good example of this. The physical movements and postures (called *asana*) range from the well-known lotus position to movements which make the body supple, tone up muscles and nerves, and improve the general working of the body.

Just as important, each posture combines mental control, and good respiration. It is necessary to move slowly and smoothly and also to breathe correctly to achieve the full benefit from the various positions. Many classes also involve exercises which concentrate the mind, rather like meditation.

Says one enthusiast with eczema: 'One of the greatest sources of relief which I have found is the regular practice of yoga, and in particular the relaxation techniques described. It is little short of miraculous how one can be free of the itch for half an hour in the *sarsana* or "corpse" position.'

Meditation can be learned at classes held in most towns now, techniques varying according to the methods used. But, basically, meditation aims to bring the mind under control, focusing on specific areas of thought and consciousness. It can also bring great peace, and practised regularly, morning and evening, can refresh both mind and body.

Some techniques are being used for specific illnesses, and visualization therapy concentrates the mind on a particular area of the body where there is disability. This is mainly used for cancer at present, but the 'mind over matter' approach might well be used to ease skin conditions like eczema.

Self-education
Relaxation classes take different forms, too, and one method used in conjunction with many branches of natural medicine is the Autogenic Relaxation Therapy. This is based on responsive conditioning induced through videos and tapes, and aims to replace negative and destructive thought processes and habits with more positive, life-enhancing ones.

The Alexander Technique is another form of self-education which corrects faulty physical habits such as bad posture and over-tense muscles, and also seeks to change patterns of behaviour and thought so that life can be lived in a more fruitful and positive way.

When eczema is very severe, people feel tempted to shut themselves away, but it's often through a new interest such as art or music or archaeology that not only do they find something to absorb themselves in mentally and physically but also find new friends.

It was after a course of acupuncture that Gillian Armstrong began to realize the part she was unwittingly playing in keeping her eczema going and decided to do something about it.

'There were three ideas that I had to accept to get well and stay well,' she writes. 'First, that the remedy to which I resort (the scratching) is the thing that is making it worse. Second, that my skin is capable of healing itself with medical help, including acupuncture and homoeopathy.

'Third, that if I will only hand the whole thing over to the healing power which I am now convinced is in the world, ready to help us if we allow it, then in my experience improvements can follow which I would not have believed possible.'

Gillian also talks about the relief she found in pouring her problems out to one person, carefully chosen as being detached, yet understanding and totally trustworthy. The support this brought allowed her to start looking at how she was handling the problems and tensions of her life.

'I discovered that I spent a great deal of time worrying about things in the future (later that day, tomorrow, next week, next year) over which I had no control. I was very good at imagining myself in a set of circumstances, and becoming more tense over my ability or otherwise to handle the imaginary situation.

'So I am learning, along with not scratching *now*, to concentrate on what I am doing *now*. Today is enough for me to handle and in fact I really enjoy life in a way which I was never able to before.'

Out in the World

Some of the things that cause worry and difficulty for people with eczema, and those who look after them, are social and environmental ones, to do with the world we live in.

From the sun in the sky, the water we drink and pollen in the air, to how other people treat and look at us, all can make a great deal of difference to a condition like this.

Though, as we've seen already, a change in attitude on the part of the person with eczema can sometimes be what is needed, in other situations the changes must be made by other people, or the solution may be quite practical.

Though the environment can at times be cruel, it is always possible to turn things to our advantage. What surrounds us can either be an enemy or a friend, depending on how we use it.

A lot, as always, will also depend on individual circumstances and attitude. But, by a process of careful detective work, you can find out what helps and what hinders, and also take steps to make the world a more comfortable place in which to live.

Water as a therapy
As we've also already seen, water is a very good example of this love/hate relationship. In certain circumstances it can do a great deal of good for people with eczema, with regular baths plus emulsifiers helping to keep the skin supple and moisturized.

Hydrotherapy also has a part to play, the special baths and water massage cleansing the pores, improving circulation and toning underlying muscle tone. Some people have wonderful results from bathing in spa waters or drinking them, others from visiting the mineral-rich waters of placed like the Dead Sea in Israel.

It is also possible to buy these minerals in packets and add them to the bath, and for some salty water is so beneficial that they use salt regularly as a part of treatment. Says one young man: 'I, like my grandmother, have suffered from eczema all my life (I am now twenty-one) and will try any remedy that is suggested. Three months ago my grandmother told me of yet another idea. At this time the eczema on my hands was extremely bad — today my hands are completely clear with no cuts and near perfect nails!

'This was achieved by soaking my hands in salt water for the first two weeks until the cuts had gone, and then, when I could bear it, rubbing salt directly into my hands day and night. The best thing is that the unbearable itching goes as soon as the salt is used.'

And says a mother: 'Quite by accident we discovered that sea-bathing cleared our daughter's skin, and so this year after our holiday we continued to bath her at home in a strong solution of *Tidman's Sea Salts* (from health stores and chemists) and she is much, much better.'

Another mother who tried homoeopathy for her daughter found that, unfortunately, the remedies did not help. But the homoeopath also recommended Epsom salts, added regularly to the bath, and this led to such improvement that it has become a part of their nightly routine.

Yet, in spite of all this, water can also be a destructive force for the sensitive skin, particularly if it is over-used and contains no soothing agents such as lubricants. Water with soap or washing up liquid and powder is especially harmful.

For some, sea water can act as an irritant, although it's true that the initial stinging and discomfort might pass after jumping in and out of the water a few times! But that can be hard on a very sore skin, especially for children. Chlorine in swimming pools is another irritant, although even that has been known as beneficial to some. It can also help to protect the skin if *Vaseline* or emulsifying ointment is smoothed into the skin before and after swimming.

Soft water suits many people better than hard water, a fact which can show itself after holidaying away from home. But before going to all the expense and trouble of installing a water softener, or even moving house, you can experiment or compromise by adding a little *Calgon* water softening powder to water run from the tap.

It's even possible to react to the contents of tap water, according to Action Against Allergy, an organization which researches and co-ordinates information in this field. One member found that when she replaced tap water with purified or bottled water, her son's skin improved beyond belief.

Climatology and eczema

Eczema sufferers are also affected by the climate they live in, the air they breathe and by the different seasons.

For some, spring, with its pollens and spores, is the worst time; for some, summer with its dry heat and harvesting; for others, autumn with moulds and damp; and for yet others winter with its frosts and cold winds. But each of these different seasons will suit other eczema sufferers perfectly!

Similarly, the climates of countries abroad will fit one person and not another. The hot and humid climate of Cyprus can be ideal, but on the other hand the sunny, dry cold of the Austrian Alps can be, too. In certain countries like Sweden, Finland and Denmark they have special centres for climatotherapy, health ministries have their own travel agencies and doctors prescribe health tours!

This may sound quite far-fetched, but it is amazing what a change of scenery can do for eczema. This may be partly to do with getting away from the usual stresses and strains of life, but in some cases it is definitely to do with the destination.

The main area for climatotherapy is around the Dead Sea. The waters of the sea contain ten times more minerals than ordinary sea water, including magnesium, the climate is dry and mild and, because the Dead Sea is below sea level, the sunlight is low in ultra-violet rays. But the climate must heal the skin before sea therapy begins, as the minerals would be too strong for a skin that is broken and sore.

Writes Margaret Minnis, who has had severe eczema for over forty years and had tried every remedy under the sun: 'I was at the end of my tether so I packed my bags and flew to Israel. Four weeks of sun and later floating in the Dead Sea wearing nothing more potent than baby oil worked the wonder that is now me! I look like a new woman.'

For some it is just the sunshine that works, and holidays in foreign countries clear up the eczema. They also benefit from sun-beds and lamps, and might find ultra-violet light treatment such as PUVA helpful. helpful.

But, at the risk of becoming extremely boring, I have to point out that the reverse can be true as well! In fact, as mentioned in the second chapter, light sensitive eczema is actually triggered or made worse by the ultra-violet rays of the sun. So sunshine, like everything else, is a matter of trial and not, I hope, too much error.

Purified air

Another problem out-of-doors can be the pollens, seeds and other airborne irritants that float around. There is an enormous variety of these and they can be extremely difficult to avoid other than by staying indoors all the time or living in an air-tight plastic bubble.

Living in the town or the country can make a difference. We definitely found that our son was affected by straw, hay and harvesting when we lived in the wilds of Norfolk, and another country holiday staying in a dusty, damp cottage in Surrey brought on every allergic reaction in the book, including asthma.

Signs as obvious as this would probably have to lead to a house move, as they did with us. But even towns can have their environmental hazards, since there are still flowers, trees and grass in gardens and parks, plus the pollution of cars and factories.

Indoors, some people find that ionizers or air purifiers which give out a mixture of electric impulses and oxygen are helpful. These also filter the air, removing dust, smoke and other possible irritants. Other types of air cleansers can be fitted to radiators, or simply plugged in and moved from room to room.

Some adults find that desensitization, the injection of small amounts of pollen or dust or whatever the offending substance is, over a period of time is successful. But this is not always the case, and at present children are mostly not thought suitable for this particular treatment, though some are being treated with the desensitization method mentioned on page 46.

So what do you do? One important answer is that perhaps by developing the generally healthier way of life outlined already in this book the body may build up a better resistance to the various irritants.

Bearing in mind that allergy and general sensitivity will be at its highest when we are at our lowest, the more fit the body is, the greater the ability to fight off the invading enemy troops — or you may simply find that the immune system ignores them altogether and gets on with more important business.

Eczema in school

Attitudes to disabilities such as eczema in schools have changed tremendously over the past few years, particularly since the report of Baroness Mary Warnock and her committee, and the 1981 Education Act.

Because of the Warnock Report and the Act there is a far greater sympathy for children with what are now called 'special needs', who include pupils with a whole range of difficulties and disabilities. It is now believed that as many as one in six children are thought to have these special needs at one time or another in their school lives.

As some of today's adult patients will remember, there was a time when children with severe eczema were either labelled 'delicate' and sent to special schools, or treated with cruel toughness in ordinary schools, often as if they were making a fuss about nothing.

One woman remembers how, in basket making classes at her convent school, she was always being given the job of holding the cane under water, even though her hands were cracked and terribly sore. Others remember being treated as untouchable by teachers as well as pupils, and being sneered at for being over-fussy because they were on a special diet.

Even though this sort of uninformed prejudice still lingers, particularly among children who have not been told the facts and adults who have not bothered to learn, the general attitude is moving much more towards understanding, acceptance and genuine integration.

Because teachers in ordinary schools are now having to cope with many more children who have disabilities, they are attending special needs courses both during initial training and once they are working in schools. Many books and articles are being published advising on the problems that can arise, emotional as well as physical.

Conditions like eczema may still be misunderstood, of course, and not all teachers and others working in education may realize just how severe the needs of a child with eczema can be. Irritation, soreness, the stigma of a rash, lack of sleep, frequent absences and difficulty in concentrating will all take their toll.

This is where the parent can play such an important role. By going in to see playgroup leaders, schoolteachers and headteachers they can point out the various problems that may arise, and possible solutions. They can also pass on helpful leaflets issued by the National Eczema Society.

In her turn, the teacher may decide to talk to the other children about the difficulties a child with eczema may have, explaining that it is not infectious but that it can cause a great deal of discomfort.

Says one eczema sufferer, now a teacher herself: 'There is a great deal that can be done at school by sensitive teachers and friendly peers. One such person intervened in my adolescent crisis and in the end I returned to school.'

Exams and careers

For the teenager with eczema, new difficulties can arise when exams and career choice come along. Unfortunately most of the important school and university exams are held at the worst time of year for eczema sufferers, when all the irritants such as pollen are at their height and the weather is usually hot and sunny.

One teenager was recently telling me how he had failed an important maths exam because it was held in a hot room with large glass windows. He became uncomfortable and itchy, lost his concentration and had to leave the room. He passed the exam when he took it again later and felt that, had he been in a more suitable setting, he would have got through first time round.

Not everyone realizes that if a letter is sent to the doctor or school medical authority explaining the situation it is possible for special facilities to be laid on and allowances made for eczema, just as for any disability or handicap. For instance, if writing is difficult because hands are sore, then a tape recorder could be used.

Career choices, for adults as well as teenagers, can also lead to much heart searching. Unfortunately, some jobs are closed to those with eczema, even though it may only affect their hands. I recently heard of a teenager barred from both army and nursing training because of her eczema, and jobs in catering present obvious difficulties.

Certain jobs, such as hairdressing, garage mechanics or work in certain types of mills or factories, may actually make the eczema worse or be causing it in the first place. As explained in the first chapter, industrial eczema is triggered by irritants and allergens commonly found at work, including oils, cements, dyes, chemicals and dust from cereals and grains.

There may be advice available from the disablement resettlement officer at the Job Centre, and if the condition is particularly serious the officer can arrange for the school-leaver to attend an employment rehabilitation centre for general assessment.

The school medical service can also help, and there are forms available which will pinpoint the sort of jobs that are not suitable, for instance in places where obvious allergens and irritants are regularly in use.

Some people choose to ignore an allergy if they want a job enough, or find some way round the problem. To fulfil an ambition and be in your chosen career can be such a comfort emotionally that this outweighs the physical difficulties, and can help the eczema improve.

In the community
Some of the practical needs associated with eczema can disrupt life quite as much as the social and emotional difficulties. For instance, the necessity for daily baths and special meals or the fact that sheets get blood-stained can make holidays or going away anywhere a problem.

There is more washing, more cleaning, more cooking for diets, more shopping as parents and adult patients look for cotton clothes and bedding, or special foods.

One mother writes of the difficulties she had living with a two-year-old suffering from severe eczema in a council flat which had underfloor heating that could not be turned off. The family asked to be rehoused, but had to endure many months of distress, with the little girl over-heated and itchy, before this eventually came about.

Another woman writes of her embarrassment about preparing food for friends when her hands are sore and scabby. Rightly or wrongly, she would feel they were put off by the sight, and eventually gave up entertaining altogether.

In the end she, like many others, found a sensible solution. In her case this was to wear rubber gloves with a cotton lining which not only made her feel more comfortable socially, but actually protected her hands from damaging agents such as washing-up water and vegetable juices.

Social workers, either attached to the local social services department or the hospital, may be able to help with other practical difficulties, from hospital fares to the lack of a bath in the home, the need for an attendance allowance or exemption from prescription charges.

Derek Gay, whose work with teenagers has already been mentioned, is one medical social worker who took his job seriously enough to see how the social, emotional and physical offshoots of eczema interweave and overlap, needing attention and counselling at all levels to put things right.

Unfortunately, not all hospitals have this type of help available, but they may be able to put patients and their families in touch with counsellors. Also, some specialists will give time to sort out difficulties which have emotional and social repercussions but may have quite physical causes.

An example of this are the sexual problems which many adults patients have in relationships, often connected with the sheer physical discomfort of the rash, the itchiness and the overheating at night, as much as low self-esteem.

It's a sad irony when this is the case, because touch and physical contact can be a great healer. As we grow older we all need to be cuddled like a child sometimes, and one of the great joys of sexual relationships is the close and loving physical warmth that one person can give to another. So something that could actually help the eczema may be denied *because* of it.

Sometimes eczema may be affecting the genital region very severely and, quite apart from general physical contact, this makes intercourse painful rather than enjoyable. The tension arising from such conflicts within a partnership can then make the problem — and the eczema — worse than ever.

Rather than leaving this, perhaps because of embarrassment at seeing the doctor over such an intimate matter, it is important to seek help. Sometimes the solution can be very simple. For instance, eczema of the genital region may actually be made worse by the very treatments that have been prescribed for it, such as strong steroids which should not be used on sensitive areas of skin.

It is also possible for rubber contraceptives, spermicides, nylon underclothing, sanitary protection, talcs, soaps, bath preparations, deodorants and even toilet paper to act as an irritant or allergen, particularly if the eczema is actually the contact type.

The rash could also be something of a different nature altogether, such as thrush (*candida*) which needs quite separate treatment from the eczema. So it is important to have a proper diagnosis and not just put up with such discomfort as part of the condition.

People with eczema need the warmth, comfort and excitement of sexual love just as much — if not more — than anyone else, and for the rash to prevent this seems a double injustice. The support and understanding of a partner is also especially important, so if practical steps don't help, then guidance should be sought from a marriage guidance sex therapist or counsellor.

Self-help

It's information of the sort talked about in this chapter and also throughout this book that self-help organizations such as the National Eczema Society can pass on in such abundance. Either through meeting fellow families and patients, attending meetings or reading the literature, knowledge grows all the time.

Through joining the Society some have discovered diet helps them or the dust mite doesn't, or for the first time have learned about something as basic as adding emulsifying ointment or oil to the bath.

But apart from helping themselves and each other, members find that there are other, wider aspects to the work of self-help groups. For instance, they can raise money for more research so that at least some of the mysteries concerning the causes and cure of eczema may be resolved.

There are projects going on all over the country at various hospitals and centres, and a research fellowship looking into various aspects of children's eczema has been funded by NES at the Institute of Child Health.

Another wider task is educating the world at large. If those who suffer from eczema and those who look after them band together they have a much better chance of educating others about the condition and what it's like to live with.

In fact, in recent years newspaper articles, television and radio programmes and magazines features have repeatedly focused on eczema, a subject which many used to think rather too down-beat and unpalatable to dwell on. This is largely due to the concerted publicity campaigns of the NES.

Members can also press for improvements in all areas of treatment, and two successful campaigns have been for washing powders to suit eczema sufferers, and for better instructions and labelling to go out with steroid preparations.

But, of course, self-help does not just work for groups, it works for individuals, too. Particularly through the use of the various natural therapies with their accent on partnership with the practitioner and personal responsibility, many more people are realizing that their health, to a large extent, lies in their own hands.

It is no longer necessary for parents or adult patients to feel totally at the mercy of the eczema, but instead we can find positive ways of putting ourselves in charge. I hope this book has at least given a starting point from which to launch this journey.

Further Reading and Useful Organizations

Chapter 1

Exchange: quarterly magazine of the National Eczema Society. Back copies available with articles from specialists, and lay people. Free to members.

National Eczema Society: Organization to help patients with eczema and their families cope with this condition. There are around fifty local groups who hold meetings, fund-raising events and social activities, and there are national conferences, children's holidays, press campaigns, counselling and various other services. Literature includes leaflets on many aspects of eczema, and details of these, plus membership, are available from NES at Tavistock House North, Tavistock Square, London WC1H 9SR. Tel: 01-388 4097.

Chapter 2

Essentials of Dermatology, by Dr John L. Burton, published by Churchill Livingstone.

Infection and Eczema plus other leaflets on types of eczema available from National Eczema Society (address above).

Chapter 3

Skin Care, leaflet available from National Eczema Society.

Diseases of Civilisation, by Brain Inglis, published by Hodder and Stoughton.

Your Child with Eczema, by David Atherton, published by Heinemann Medical Books.

Chapter 4

Allergies: Questions and Answers, by Dr A. W. Franklin and Dr D. Rapp, published by Heinemann Medical Books.

Hyperactive Children's Support Group: Has information, recipes, leaflets helpful to children — and adults — suffering from a wide range of allergic reactions. Details from 59 Meadowside, Angmering, Sussex BN16 4BW.

National Society for Research into Allergy: Organization co-ordinating and encouraging research into many aspects of allergy, behavioural as well as physical. Details from PO Box 45, Hinckley, Leicestershire, LE10 1JY.

Action Against Allergy: Another campaigning organization pushing for more information and better treatments for allergic conditions. Contact AAA at 43 The Downs, London SW20 8HG. Tel: 01-947-5082.

American Allergy Association: Has regular newsletter with information on discoveries and developments worldwide. Details from PO Box 7273, Mento Park, California 94026.

Cotton On: Mail order firm selling cotton clothes. Write to 29 North Clifton Street, Lytham FY8 5HW. Tel: 0253-736611.

Clothes for Children, a leaflet from National Eczema Society with more useful addresses, including sources of cotton blankets.

Chapter 5

Dietary Treatment of Eczema, a diet information pack, available from National Eczema Society.

Not All In the Mind by Dr Richard Mackarness published by Pan Books.

Foresight: The Association for Promotion of Pre-conceptual Care, has useful literature and can be contacted at The Old Vicarage, Church Lane, Witley, Surrey GU8 5PN. Tel: Wormley (042879) 4900.

National Childbirth Trust, 9 Queensborough Terrace, London W2 3TB. Tel: 01-221-3833; *La Leche League,* PO Box 3424, London WC1V 6XX; and *Association of Breastfeeding Mothers,* 131 Mayon Road, London SE26. All have local groups and guidance to help with successful breastfeeding.

The Allergy Diet, by Elizabeth Workman S.R.D., Dr John Hunter and Dr Virginia Alun Jones, published by Dunitz.

Allergy? Think About Food, by Susan Lewis, published by Wisebuy, London.

Chapter 6

What Can I Give Him Today? by Diana Wells S.R.N., price 85p inc. post, is available from the author, 19a Parton Road, Churchdown, Glos. GL3 2AB.

British Goat Society, Rougham, Bury St Edmunds, Suffolk IP30 9LJ. Tel: Beyton (0359) 70351, and the *British Sheep Dairying Association,* Wield Wood, Nr Alresford, Hants SO24 9RV. Tel: Alton (0420) 63151. Both can provide literature and names and addresses of local breeders and milk suppliers.

Milk Allergy Self Help: A group specifically helping those with milk intolerance. Details from 4 Queen Anne's Grove, Bush Hill Park, Enfield, Middlesex. Tel: 01-360-2348.

Wheat-free, Milk-free, Egg-free Cooking, by Rita Greer, published by Thorsons.

E for Additives, by Maurice Hanssen, lists all the 'E' numbers for preservatives, colourings and other additives and gives details of the foods you'll find them in. Published by Thorsons.

Look at the Label also lists 'E' numbers and is available from Ministry of Agriculture, Fisheries and Food Publications Unit, Lion House, Willowburn Trading Estate, Alnwick, Northumberland NE66 2PF.

Food Additives is a leaflet explaining what additives are for, and is available from Food and Drink Industries Council, 25 Victoria Street, London SW1 0EX. Tel: 01-222-1533.

Henry Doubleday Research Association, Department FF, Convent Lane, Bocking, Braintree, Essex CM7 6RW. Tel: Braintree 0376-24083; *Organic Growers Association,* Aeron Park, Llangeithe, Dyfed. Tel Llangeithe (097423) 272; and *The Soil Association,* Walnut Tree Manor, Haughley, Stowmarket, Suffolk IP14 3RS. Tel: Haughley (044970) 235. Can all give information on organic growing, free from pesticides and other contamination.

Foodwatch: Specializes in supplying pure foods, plus technical advice on labelling, food composition, etc. Contact them at High Acre, East Stour, Gillingham, Dorset SP8 55R. Tel: 0747-85261.

Free Range Egg Association: Will, in return for a large S.A.E. send list of shops that supply free range eggs. Write to FREGG at 37 Tanza Road, London NW3 2UA.

Camhealth, 7 Castle Street, Tonbridge, Kent. Tel: 0732-364546; *McCarrison Society,* 23 Stanley Court, Worcester Road, Sutton, Surrey SM2 65D. Tel: 01-643-2812; and *British Nutrition Foundation,* 15 Belgrave Square, London SW1X 8PS. Tel: 01-235-4904. All campaign for better food quality and healthier diets.

Vegan Society Has useful information, including recipes, on vegan diet. Write to PO Box 3, Charlbury, Oxford OX7 6DU. Tel: (0993) 831470.

Vegetarian Society: Has similar guide lines on following a vegetarian diet. Write to 53 Marloes Road, London W8 6LA. Tel: 01-937-7739.

Community Health Foundation: Has information on the macrobiotic diet. Send for leaflets to 188 Old Street, London EC1V 9BP. Tel: 01-251-4076.

Coeliac Society: Provides information on gluten-free diet and sources of gluten-free products. Write to PO Box 181, London NW2 2QY.

Hyperactive Children's Support Group: Particularly helpful on additive-free diets, and can supply diet sheets and recipes to members. Write to address given under Chapter 4 section.

Chapter 7

Natural Health Network: Links many natural health centres in various parts of the country. Write to the network at Chardstock House, Chard, Somerset. Tel: Chard (04606) 3229.

Institute for Complementary Medicine: Can give details of your nearest information point on alternative therapies. Write to them at 21 Portland Place, London W1N 3AF. Tel: 01-636-9543.

Council for Complementary and Alternative Medicine: Provides a forum for communication and co-operation, plus high standards of training, for various therapies. Details from 10 Belgrave Square, London SW1X 8PH. Tel: 01-235-9512.

Radionics Association: The professional body for those who practise radionics. List of practitioners is available from them at 16a North Bar, Banbury, Oxfordshire OX16 0TF. Tel: Banbury (0295) 3183.

British Society of Dowsers: Can give information on this therapy and also local practitioners. Contact the Society at Sycamore Cottage, Tamley Lane, Hastingleigh, Ashford, Kent TN25 5HW. Tel: 0233-75 253.

Chapter 8

British Naturopathic and Osteopathic Association, Frazer House, 6 Netherhall Gardens, London NW3 5RR. Tel: 01-453-8728; *British Register of Naturopaths,* 1 Albermarle Road, The Mount, York YO2 1EN. Tel: York (0904) 23693; and *The Osteopathic and Naturopathic Guild,* 18 Elgin Road, Talbot Woods, Bournemouth, Dorset BN4 9NL. Tel: Bournemouth (0202) 769297. All can supply names of qualified practitioners.

The General Council and Register of Osteopaths: Has register of qualified practitioners. Write to the Council at 1-4 Suffolk Street, London SW1Y 4MG. Tel: 01-839-2060.

British Chiropractic Association: Has a register of members who have graduated from recognized colleges. Write for details to 5 First Avenue, Chelmsford, Essex CM1 1RX. Tel: Chelmsford (0245) 358487.

Health Stores Handbook published by the National Association of Health Stores gives information on nature cure clinics and other forms of natural therapy, and health foods. Copies available from N.A.H.S. at Queens Road, Nottingham NG2 3AS. Tel: Nottingham (0602) 474165.

Vitalax and other naturopathic remedies are available from Healthwise, 11 Plains Road, Mapperley, Nottingham.

Bran and Other Natural Aids for Intestinal Fitness, by Ray Hill, published by Thorsons.

Chapter 9

The Home Herbal, by Barbara Griggs published by Jill Norman and Hobhouse.

Nature's Plan for Your Health, by Thomas Bartram, giving guidance on the use of herbs and many other aspects of natural medicine, published by Blandford Press. Thomas Bartram is also editor of the magazine *Grace.*

National Institute of Medical Herbalists, 41 Hatherley Road, Winchester, Hants SO22 6RR. Tel: Winchester (0962) 68776; *The British Herbal Medicine Association,* Lane House, Cowling, Keighley, West Yorkshire BD22 0LX. Tel: Cross Hills (0535) 34487; and *The Herb Society,* 34 Boscobal Place, London SW1. Tel: 01-235-1023. All can supply information on herbalism and on qualified practitioners.

Evening Primrose Oil, by Judy Graham, published by Thorsons.

Bach Flower Remedies: Information is available from the Edward Bach Centre, Mount Vernon, Sotwell, Wallingford, Oxon OX10 0PZ. Tel: Wallingford (0491) 39489.

Chapter 10

The Homoeopathic Development Foundation, 19a Cavendish Square, London W1M 9AD. Tel: 01-629-3205; *British Homoeopathic Association,* 27a Devonshire Street, London W1N 1RJ. Tel: 01-935 2163; *The Society of Homoeopaths,* 101 Sebastian Avenue, Shenfield, Brentwood, Essex CM15 8PP; and *The Hahnemann Society,* Humane Education Centre, Avenue Lodge, Bounds Green Road, London N22 4EU. Tel: 01-889-1595 can all supply information on homoeopathy and in, most cases, names of practitioners. Treatment is also available on the National Health Service and The British Homoeopathic Association can provide names of hospitals and practitioners.

Homoeopathy Today is a magazine published by The Hahnemann Society.

New Era Laboratories: Have a hair analysis service, and can also supply information on tissue salts. Details from New Era Laboratories, Dept BH, 39 Wales Farm Road, London W3 6XH. Tel: 01-992-8656.

Chapter 11

British Acupuncture Association, 34 Alderney Street, London SW1V 4EU. Tel: 01-834-1012; *Traditional Acupuncture Society,* 11 Grange Park, Stratford-upon-Avon, Warwickshire CV37 6XH. Tel: 0789 298798; and the *Register of Traditional Chinese Medicine* 7A Thorndean Street, London SW18 4HE. Tel: 01-947-1879. All can give information on acupuncture and allied methods, plus qualified practitioners.

Shiatsu Society: Can give information on this therapy, and is at 3 Elia Street, London N1. Tel: 01-278-6783.

International Institute of Reflexology: Trains reflexologists and has names of registered practitioners. Contact them at PO Box 34, Harlow, Essex CM17 0LT. Tel: Harlow (0279) 29060.

Touch for Health: There are local training courses and therapists and for more information write to British Touch for Health Association, 37-39 Brondesbury Road, London NW3.

Chapter 12

Tavistock Clinic arranges both family, group and individual therapy with skilled people, and should also be able to put you in touch with counsellors in other areas of the country. Write to the Tavistock Clinic, Belsize Lane, London NW3.

British Hypnotherapy Association, 67 Upper Berkeley Street, London W1. Tel: 01-723-4443; and the *British Society of Medical and Dental Hypnosis,* 42 Links Road, Ashtead, Surrey KT21 2HJ. Both can give names of qualified practitioners and information on the therapy.

The National Federation of Spiritual Healers, Old Manor Farm Studio, Church Street, Sunbury-on-Thames, Middlesex TW16 6RG. Tel: Sunbury (09327) 83164; and *The Aetherius Society* 757 Fulham Road, London SW6 5UU. Tel: 01-736-4187 both seek to increase knowledge and understanding of spiritual healing. They may be able to put you in touch with suitable centres.

British Wheel of Yoga, 80 Leckhampton Road, Cheltenham, Gloucestershire GL53 0BN. Tel: Cheltenham (0242) 524889; and *Friends of Yoga,* 5 Weston Crescent, Old Sawley, Long Eaton, Nottingham NG10 3BS. Tel: Long Eaton (0602) 735435. Both have register of qualified teachers and can provide information on yoga.

Autogenic Relaxation Therapy: For more details of this write to *British Association for Autogenic Training and Therapy,* 101 Harley Street, London W1. Tel: 01-935-1811.

Society of the Alexander Technique: Has directory of recognized teachers. Write to 3b Albert Court, Kensington Gore, London SW7. Tel: 01-584-3834.

London School of Aromatherapy, has list of qualified therapists and can be contacted at 42a Hillfield Park, London N10.

Chapter 13

VIP Health Holidays: Arrange trips for eczema sufferers to the Dead Sea in Israel. For details write to 42 Audley Street, London W1A 4PY. Tel: 01-499-4221.

Finders Dead Sea Health: Can give details of Dead Sea mineral salts. Write to Freepost, Cranbrook, TN17 3BR or for free advice telephone 0580-713603.

British Association of Art Therapists, 13c Northwood Road, London N6 5LT. Tel: 01-348-6143; and *British Society for Music Therapy,* Guildhall School of Music and Drama, Barbican, London EC2Y 8DT. Tel: 01-368-8879. Both promote art and music as a form of therapy. For details of therapists, write to them.

Coping at School is a leaflet from the National Eczema Society useful to both parents and teachers.

Ionizers: For information contact Medion Ltd., Box 1, Oxted, Surrey or The London Ioniser Centre, 67 Endell Street, London WC2H 9AJ.

Index

(Please note: Under headings such as adults, children, etc. the index lists pages referring specifically to this group. However, general advice given throughout the book on aspects of eczema will be appropriate for all age groups.)